Pran

The Yoga

ANDRÉ VAN LYSEBETH

By the same author:

Yoga Self-taught
Tantra: The Cult of the Feminine

Harmony Publishing
25 Rodney Street
Edinburgh
EH7 4EL
Scotland
www.harmonypublishing.org
contact@harmonypublishing.org

First published in Great Britain by Unwin Paperbacks 1979
This edition: 2007
Printed and bound in Korea
ISBN 978-0-9552412-3-9

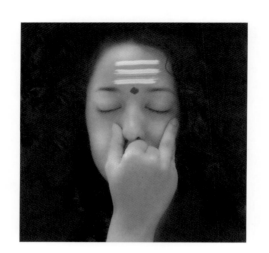

Contents

PART THREE: ESOTERIC PRANAYAMA, ITS BASES AND ITS PRACTICE

Part 1

WHAT IS PRANA?
WHAT DOES SCIENCE THINK OF IT?

1 | What is Prana?

Prana is to yoga what electricity is to modern civilisation. Let us suppose for a moment that we have been taken back by time machine into the presence of a yogi of two thousand years ago and that we are trying to explain to him what our own way of life is like, with its aeroplanes, telephone, radio, television, refrigerators, motor cars, vacuum cleaners, satellites and space rockets, electronic brains, pocket lamps, tramcars and food mixers - but without mentioning electricity. The view he would get of our civilisation would be very false indeed, for he would understand nothing of its basic driving force, the electricity which we use without thinking much about it except in the event of a power failure.

In the same way, to be ignorant of Prana, or not to appreciate its existence and its influence on our bodies, how to store it and direct it at will, is to be ignorant of the true yoga. Of course it is possible to practise the asanas without being involved with prana, because to some extent the postures almost automatically ensure pranic balance even though the adept is little concerned with it. But after a certain period of such practise he reaches a limit. Once the technique of the postures is acquired the adept must go on beyond the stage of purely mechanical and material execution of the asanas and similar yogic exercises if he is to reach the state of Pranayama.

First of all, like the Indian philosophers, we must define the terms we are going to use.

What is Prana?
So what is Prana? Is it some mysterious occult force, the source of miraculous power?

According to Swami Sivananda, 'Prana is the sum total of all the energy in the universe.' This is surely something vast! For the yogis the universe is composed of Akasa, the cosmic ether, and Prana, energy. When Prana acts upon Akasa all forms of matter are created. This idea corresponds broadly to that of modern nuclear physics, which regards all matter as energy 'organised' in different ways. But our science does not admit (or no longer admits) the notion of ether, at least for the time being.

Prana with a capital P designates the cosmic energy in its entirety, while prana with a small p indicates its manifestations. Thus Prana is undifferentiated universal energy, while prana is the differentiated energy revealed in every possible form. Magnetism is a manifestation of Prana, so are electricity and gravitation. Everything in the universe that moves is a manifestation of Prana; thanks to Prana the wind blows, the earth trembles, an axe falls, an aeroplane takes off, a star explodes, a philosopher thinks. We exist in an ocean of Prana where every living thing is a vortex. Yogis affirm that what characterises life is its ability to attract Prana to itself, to store it up and transform it for influence upon both the inner and outer world.

It might be asked why the term Prana is used rather than 'energy'. For Westerners the term 'energy', however, is too broad and too materialistic. For the yogi thought itself is a more subtle form of prana, while for the Westerner energy is something fundamentally different. Our word 'energy' is, shall we say, too industrial. According to the yogis, it is present in the air, yet it is neither oxygen, nor nitrogen, nor any other chemical constituent of the atmosphere. Prana exists in our food, water, sunlight, but it is neither vitamin nor warmth nor ultraviolet rays. Air, water, food, sunlight: all convey the prana on which all animal and vegetable life depends. Prana penetrates the whole body, even where the air cannot reach. Prana is our true nourishment, for without prana there can be no life. Vitality itself is no more than a special and subtle form of prana, which fills the whole universe. To make itself manifest on the material plane the spirit uses prana to animate the body and its organs.

So far we have not seriously attacked modern Western ideas, but the yogis go beyond an affirmation of the existence of this energy, an energy which no nuclear physicist would deny. For the rishis proclaim — and this forms the very basis of yoga — that prana can be stored in the nervous system, more particularly in the solar plexus. Furthermore, they emphasise this cardinal and essential idea that yoga gives us the power, through thought, of directing the current of prana at will. Yoga thus gives us conscious and voluntary access to the very sources of life.

Conscious control of prana

To reveal the existence of prana is remarkable; but to discover that it can be controlled and to fix the laws and techniques to that end is marvellous and the yogis have done both. The science of controlling prana is called pranayama (*ayama* = to curb or to master). All yoga exercises, not only the respiratory techniques, have that in view; for example, by controlling prana the yogis can stop their hearts from beating.

Experiments have been carried out on the spot in India by Dr Thérèse Brosse, with simultaneous pneumographic and cardio-graphic recordings, and here is an extract from her published report:

'Just when the yogi announces that his heart is under control only the minutest fibrillation is visible on the iso-electric graph, the merest trace of cardiac contraction and almost impossible to record. On seeing this trace it would be possible to reach the most serious prognosis were it not that, in the moments immediately before and after, the recorded line is not only normal but even exaggerated in voltage at the will of the yogi.

'Faced with such facts it is of little importance that we attribute them to an abnormal concentration of carbon dioxide in the blood, to a change of the heart's axis, to a modification of tissue ionisation, to a combination of all these processes or others unsuspected of which the present state of our knowledge does not permit us to take account. Whatever it might be it remains truly astonishing that the extreme fall in voltage takes place precisely when the yogi announces that he is about to withdraw the vital energy from his heart, and that the voltage returns to normal or above it when he claims that he is in control of the normal functioning of his heart. To the mind of the yogi the vital energy (prana) is an electrical energy which he declares is of the same nature as lightning. On the other hand it is by a special science of breathing that he means to regulate that vital energy, at least that which he draws from nature. Quite recent works have made clear the role of the lungs so far as the electrical charge in the blood is con-cerned, the alveoli extracting the negative ions from the inhaled air, which pass on their vitality to the colloids.

'Thus we find ourselves in the presence of men with an almost com-plete mastery of the various human activities and who, without any knowledge of the structure of their organs, can master their functions nonetheless. Moreover, they enjoy magnificent health which they could not maintain if they were ceaselessly violating physiological laws during their extraordinary and prolonged exercises. As we have just seen, the very theory on which some of these exercises are based seems to be confirmed, not only by the results but also by recent discoveries by Western science.'

To interpret 'pranayama' as 'breathing exercises' would be to limit sadly the scope of the exercises and to misunderstand their true purpose, which is the collecting, storing and conscious control of the vital pranic energies in our bodies. In the final analysis pranayama is also the goal of the asanas, bandhas and mudras; between the mental level and prana there is an interaction which ensures that Hatha yoga is something more than physical. Indeed, between mental yoga or Raja yoga and Hatha yoga there is no fundamental difference.

To sum up: Prana is the sum total of the energy of the universe. Prana is neither magnetism, nor gravitation, nor electricity, though these various phenomena are all manifestations of the universal Prana. Prana is manifest everywhere in the universe where there is movement. The most delicate of movements like those of the electrons round the atomic nucleus or the muscular force of a brutal punch are all manifestations of the universal Prana. Life, the 'life force', is a manifestation of Prana like the rest.

To end this first section here are a few paragraphs from de Hufeland's *The Art of Prolonging the Life of Man*, published early in the nineteenth century, which contains ideas astonishingly close to the yogic ideas discussed above:

'What is life? What is the vital force? These questions are among the many we encounter at every step in our study of nature. Apparently simple, they arise from only very ordinary phenomena, facts which we observe every day; yet they are very difficult to answer. As soon as a philosopher uses the word "force" one may be sure that he is in trouble, for he is trying to explain something by a word which is itself an enigma. In fact, has anyone until now given a clear idea of what this word "force" means? Nevertheless, in the science of physics we have seen the introduction of an infinite number of "forces", for instance gravitation, attraction, electricity, magnetism, and so forth, which basically are none other than the x of algebra, the great unknown quantity we are seeking. However, we do need signs to represent those things of which we cannot deny the existence but whose essence is incomprehensible…

'The vital force is undeniably one of the most general, most powerful and most incomprehensible in nature. It fills and moves everything. It is probably the source of every other force in the physical world, producing, preserving and renewing everything; for thousands of years, every spring, restoring to us the brilliance and freshness of creation just as it left the hands of the Creator. It is inexhaustible and infinite like the true breath of divinity. This, perfected and exalted by a more perfect organisation, is what animates the sources of mind and spirit and gives to each reasonable being not only its existence but also the feeling for and enjoyment of life, for I have always observed that the feeling one has of the value and happiness of existence is more or less related to the strength of the vital force, and that, just as a certain superabundance of life increases our participation in all pleasures and activities, and helps us to find a greater charm in living, so nothing is more likely to produce the distaste for life and the boredom that characterises our century than a lack of the vital force. A careful study of the phenomena of the vital force in the organised world leads us to recognise in it the following properties and laws: the vital force is the most subtle, most penetrating, most invisible agent we have known until now in nature; in this respect it surpasses even light, electricity and magnetism, with which in other respects it seems to have the greatest analogy. Although it enters into every body, there are however certain forms of matter for which it seems to have greater affinity than for others; it unites with them more intimately and in greater quantity, and seems to identify itself with them. This form of matter we call "organic structure" — or simply organisation — and we describe as "organised" all bodies which possess it, that is the vegetable world and the animal world. This organic structure seems constituted in a certain way, of a certain mixture of the most delicate particles, and in this respect we find a striking analogy between the vital force and magnetism. The life force can exist in a free or latent state, and in this respect has a close analogy to heat and electricity.'

These lines are taken, let it be emphasised, from a French translation published in 1838!

2 | P r a n a   o f   t h e   A i r

The most important source of vital prana is the atmosphere. Several thousands of years before our scientists identified electricity the yogis had revealed that the atmosphere vibrates with a subtle energy and that this energy is the main source of all the other kinds of energy active in the human body. In this connection a most significant statement is the one from Dr Thérèse Brosse quoted in the previous section, in which a yogi says that 'the energy which allows him to control his heart, and even to stop it, is of the same nature as lightning'. The statement is the more surprising when we remember that lightning has always been — and still is — regarded by primitive peoples as a terrifying, even supernatural phenomenon, and that they are far from establishing an identity of nature or any relationship whatever between lightning and the vital energies which make their own organisms function.

If we relate the theories of the yogis to the observations and discoveries of Western science we can affirm that the prana in the atmosphere is composed, if not completely at least fundamentally, of electrically charged particles, negative ions in fact, and also that a true metabolism takes place within our bodies of the electricity we draw from the atmosphere. In this field Western sources are of value, though they are relatively few, since our scientists are more interested in what is going on in the Van Allen belt than in the phenomena of ionisation in the atmosphere at ground level - where we live, our vital surroundings.

For information on the subject of atmospheric electricity and its biological repercussions our choice has been limited to two research scientists working in different countries; one is Fred Vlès, professor in the Faculty of Medicine at the University of Strasbourg and Director of the Institute of Biological Physics; and the other is the Russian, Tchijewski, from Kiev. We draw mainly from the work of Vlès, particularly his fascinating book, *The Biological Conditions Created by the Electric Properties of the Atmosphere,*[*] which should have revolutionised biology but which did not arouse the general interest it deserved.

Yin and Yang
It is surprising to note that with a few rare exceptions science has failed

---

[*]   Herman & Cie, 6 rue de la Sorbonne, Paris

until quite recently to consider the influence of atmospheric electricity on the human being. Geophysicists have explained that the earth is a conductor, that its surface is charged negatively while the upper atmosphere is positive. The atmosphere, our vital environment, is situated in an approximately vertical electrostatic field with a potential gradient of between 100 and 150 volts per metre altitude. The existence of this vertical field has been known to the Chinese from antiquity.

The Chinese concept of Yin and Yang has been described as follows by Soulié de Morant, who introduced Chinese acupuncture to Europe after the First World War: 'One of the most disturbing aspects of Chinese science is the prime importance it gives to the Yin-Yang relationship. This double expression is used in many and varied senses and often confuses the research worker. Yang is what is up above in relationship to what is down below; Yang is the inverse of Yin. Ever since electricity has been known the positive pole has been named Yang and the negative Yin.

'Doctors E. and H. Biancini of Paris have assembled in an exceedingly interesting article* the scattered ideas on the relationship of atmospheric and cosmic electricity and human physiology. It is interesting to compare this with Chinese ideas on the subject.

'For the existence and signs of this energy Beccaria showed a long time ago that the normal sign when the sky is calm is positive.

'The Chinese call the positive energy Yang and attribute its origin to the sun and the stars; the negative energy is called Yin and they attribute its origin to the earth. A Chinese book of the sixteenth century presents the question in these terms:

' "Yang is what is light and pure. It is the energy which floats up high and of which the sky is made. Yin is thick and heavy. It is that which has taken shape to form the earth. The energy of the blue sky is up above, but the vegetables feed on it…"

'How could the ancient Chinese (for these ideas are reproduced from works that date from the twenty-eighth century BC) have perceived these forces and under the name Yang energy distinguished positive atmospheric electricity, and under the name of Yin energy the negative charge of the earth? We do not know.'

---

* *L'électricité atmosphérique, son rôle en biologie er en physiologie humaine'* Paris-Mecale, 15 April 1919.

Biological climatology is the basis of the ideas which are important for the understanding of yoga and of our reactions to various geographical regions and climatic conditions. For the moment we shall note only that the 'potential gradient' of the atmosphere varies considerably according to the time and place (diurnal and seasonal variations). Cosmic events influence it too: the phases of the moon, the sun's activity, etc. All meteorological factors modify it and in certain circumstances the electrical field can even be reversed temporarily.

Prana - negative ions
Let us consider the ionisation of the atmosphere. Lightning is one of its most obvious manifestations. One single flash discharges into the air the equivalent of several days' consumption of electricity by a capital city the size of Paris! However, atmospheric electricity is always important, even when it does not appear in the spectacular form of lightning.

First of all remember that an ion is an electrically charged atom or fragment of a molecule and that the ions are the workers of life in the cell. In the atmosphere there are two types of ions:

(*a*) The small negative or normal ions; very active electrically, they are minute packets of electrical energy in an almost pure state. In the air we breathe they are usually formed of one or several oxygen or nitrogen atoms and they carry a charge which corresponds to a single electron. These small negative ions bring vitality to the organism: they represent atmospheric prana in its active form.
(*b*) The large or slow ions, formed of a polymolecular nucleus, therefore much greater, to which a normal negative ion is added - one might rather say has been trapped by the large nucleus.

Remember then that the small, vitalising, negative ions are fast and very mobile while the large, slow ions play the part of a fly trap, gluing together the small ions which they attract and catch in passing. The presence of numerous large, slow ions formed through the capture of small and very mobile ions diminishes the conductivity of the air, which is what happens when the air is polluted with dust, smoke or fog. Roughly speaking, the concentration of small ions in the atmosphere diminishes when the number of large ones increases and vice versa, and the concentration of the one is in inverse proportion to the other.

That is why there is a superabundance of large ions in the dirty atmosphere of cities. In the country, where the air is clean, there are two or three small ions for each large one, whereas in the town the proportion is one small one for 275 large ones and in some cases for 600 large ones! If we consider the negative ions as 'the workers of life inside the cell' (Dr Goust), we can understand to what extent the atmosphere of the towns is poor in prana and therefore debilitating.

These facts explain and confirm the yogic theories which state that prana is neither oxygen nor nitrogen nor any other chemical constituent of the atmosphere, for in town or country the proportion of oxygen in the atmosphere is the same. It is the predominance of large, slow ions which makes the air of big towns less stimulating and revivifying. Consequently dust is at least as harmful as car exhaust gases and industrial fumes, as it absorbs and neutralises all the atmospheric prana. Yet the air-conditioning of our apartments does not restore the small negative ions. The only solution is to prevent the dust from coming into the atmosphere before it empties it of the small vitalising ions. Smoke and fog act in the same way and in our towns these three factors play the same role. Is it surprising, therefore, that the Londoner's vitality* diminishes considerably during the winter? This point will be discussed in the next section.

Sources of small vitalising ions
To ionise oxygen atoms negatively means adding electrical energy. This will only take place under the influence of important sources of energy. Telluric radiation, that is to say the natural radioactive emanations of the earth which are so weak that they do us no harm, as opposed to artificial radioactivity which is far more powerful, are an important factor in the ionisation of the air (certain rocks send out gamma rays). However, the main source of vitalising negative ions consists of short-wave electromagnetic radiations from that inexhaustible generator of electricity, the sun.

Cosmic rays are another source. These are very important, for while the sun's rays are intermittent (because of the alternation of day and night and interference by the cloud screen) cosmic rays are active continuously. They penetrate the thickest layers of cloud without losing any of their energy; they can even be found in the ground.

---

* London's air is now much less polluted following strong measures which have been taken. It is a good sign that the swallows are returning to nest in the city.

Enormous quantities of vitalising ions are produced by great masses of water in movement or in the course of evaporation; this is why sea air is so vitalising, not only because of the presence of iodine, which plays only a minor part. Beside the sea all the conditions for maximum vitalising ionisation are brought together: great masses of water in movement and evaporation, the action of the wind from the sea, the absence of dust, maximum ionisation by the sun and cosmic rays. On the coast and at sea we bathe in an ocean of prana, which is sometimes even too strong for certain ultra-sensitive organisms, incapable of absorbing and using a rush of superabundant energy. Some children become nervous and irritable; some adults cannot sleep. One of the aims of pranayama, amongst others, is to enable us to fix more of this energy, to store it, to distribute it within the organism, and to direct it wherever the need is felt.

These theoretical considerations lead directly to practice. 'An ounce of practice,' said Swami Sivananda, 'is better than tons of theory.'

The metabolism of electricity
Metabolism usually means the totality of the transformations effected by our bodies upon the food molecules we absorb either to build up the cell structures or to release vital energy. There is also a water metabolism which acts as maid of all work in the body. It forms the intra- or extracellular fluid, then enters into the composition of blood and lymph, etc., and finally dissolves the toxic substances in order to eliminate them through the skin, lungs, intestines and kidneys. However, we do not usually realise that a real metabolism of electricity also exists, and Vlès's great merit is his study of this process. An animal — and this term includes man – becomes negatively charged by the absorption of small negative ions. These follow a complicated path through the organism and participate in redox processes.[*] All vital phenomena are accompanied by oxidation or reduction as well as other roles and actions which are much more complex and take place inside the cell, especially the nerve cells. The other metabolisms are in some way dependent on this electric metabolism. A mammal in its natural state ingests the negative charges from the inhaled oxygen until satura-

---

[*]   The addition of an electron corresponds to a reduction and its removal to an oxidation.

tion is reached and eliminates the excess by general leakage through the skin. Like our car batteries we must put ourselves on charge in order to saturate ourselves with negative electricity and let the skin evacuate any excess. Vlès found that when charged to the same degree a dead mouse discharges itself very slowly whereas a live mouse shows a strong loss of negative energy, an indication of intense vital electrical activity. This indicates that the organism is well provided with small, vitalising, negative ions. Thus Western science joins and entirely confirms the yogic theories about prana.

Vlès has established that warm-blooded animals, and therefore all mammals, have a greater loss of electricity than cold-blooded animals such as the frog, where the loss is almost zero. For the mammal, which is able to regulate temperature, the process of electrical exchange with the atmosphere is thus very important. The frog depends less than we do on atmospheric prana. The metabolism of electricity, measurable and measured, explains many things. The assimilation of negative ions has to be very great in order to keep the living organism at its maximum activity, to charge the batteries fully, and to assure elimination of used ions, since the body needs to renew its charges continuously and actively. Electrically, the healthy body can be compared to a mountain lake continuously fed with fresh water which runs out at the same rate through a stream, whereas a sickly body is like a bog where the water stagnates and becomes foul. The loss of ions appears to be as important as their intake.

Encouraging the electrical metabolism
Vlès has shown that this discharge of electricity is helped by the photochemical action of ultraviolet light, which comes notably from the sun's rays. Sunbathing vitalises us by activating our electrical metabolism. This is why the body must not be electrically insulated, why it should be in contact with the earth in order to permit a constant electrical discharge. In nature all animals, according to Fabre's fanciful expression, 'undergo permanent electrotherapy' without being able to avoid it. The fur holds the air trapped between its hairs and constitutes the best thermal insulation without interfering with the elimination of electricity. On the contrary, the hairs act like lightning conductors in reverse. We have all of us observed the electricity in a cat's fur; when we stroke the cat we can hear the crackle of the static. Through their

feet the animals have direct contact with the earth; in fact, their organism is earthed. This process is so important that Vlès questions the value of much of the research on mammalian metabolism conducted on caged animals without taking electrical conditions into account. With humans clothing forms an insulating layer which restricts the normal discharge of electricity through the skin and reduces electrical exchanges with the atmosphere. Moreover, it stops the ultraviolet rays. Our shoes insulate us electrically and thus contribute to the reduction of our vitality. Tribes who go about naked or with little clothing have always had much greater vitality; as soon as they begin to dress, following the example of the whites, their vitality declines. The Western suits which African Negroes adopt are nonsensical and have a detrimental effect on their health.

Thus the idea of prana in the form of atmospheric electricity and the need for its constant renewal explains why walking barefoot in nature produces a particular sense of well-being which is not felt on the parquet flooring of a room, where the organism functions without an 'earth'. Kneipp, who seems to have known this by intuition, had recommended walking barefoot in the dew-soaked grass of morning. The dew favours 'earthing the body'. Walking barefoot in a river or stream has an effect which bathing the feet in a basin cannot give. A study of the pranic aspect of certain phenomena clarifies many mysterious and seemingly inexplicable facts and suggests practical applications, not only for our general behaviour but especially for yogic breathing.

Sauna and prana

An unexpected aspect of the phenomenon is the sauna. In fact Vlès agrees that an animal which charges itself negatively by absorbing negative ions through breathing can perhaps also do so by shedding positive ions through the evaporation of water. Now if there is one place propitious for abundant evaporation it is surely the sauna. After a good sauna bath one feels as dynamic and 'recharged' as after a long walk in the country, and this cannot be the consequence of the elimination of toxins alone. The opening of the capillaries and the increase in the circulation of the blood all over the body lead to a general toning up which can to a large extent explain the effects of the sauna. Yet the feeling of 'recharge' and of 'dynamism' can also stem from an increase in the electrical charge of the organism.

3 | Prana and Climate

Chemically the air is a simple gaseous mixture of approximately 20 per cent oxygen, 78 per cent nitrogen and 1 per cent argon, with other rarer gases. Whereas on the surface of the globe its composition is physically remarkably constant, electrically it is very variable. From one moment to the next and from one place to another its properties change considerably and are sometimes even reversed.

Geographical variations are of primary importance as they can influence some of our most important decisions, varying from the choice of where to spend a holiday to where to build a house.

The atmosphere - a prana-impregnated ocean - is not uniformly saturated with prana: it has its calm zones and its turbulent regions, its currents and lakes, its visible and invisible storms, like the magnetic storms which interest man largely because they disturb radio com-munications rather than because of their repercussions on human health. As soon as one studies these subtle pranic phenomena, matters like barometric pressure, rainfall or snowfall, strength and direction of the wind, and humidity of the air, all take second place from the viewpoint of vitality.

There are important differences between the various geographical regions, and man did not wait till the twentieth century before noticing the beneficial effect of the climate of certain places, such as the seaside or high mountains. Man searched long for an explanation in the purely chemical properties of the atmosphere of such places: for example, the revitalising effect of a stay on the Atlantic coast was attributed to the iodine and bromine vapours from the sea, to the salt in the air and to the presence of silica on the sandy beaches. These elements play a part, doubtless, as does the presence of oligo-elements whose importance from a hygienic and therapeutic point of view is only now beginning to show itself and to open up vast perspectives. Indeed, as scientific research advances the physical properties of the air become more and more important. The physiological changes caused by the climate are often immediate. The city dweller at the coast is either overcome by sleep or becomes too excited to sleep, depending on his nature. The physical properties of the air have much to do with this.

The electrical field of the atmosphere
The electrical field of the atmosphere - not to be confused with ionisation - was until very recently known only to meteorologists; biologists
were not interested. The 'electrical field' must not be confused with
the 'negative ions' already described. The difference in potential per
metre of altitude is what we are now going to discuss; it is called the
'potential gradient'. The earth is an electrified sphere whose voltage
varies greatly with altitude, with differences of up to 100 volts per
metre. In some cases the potential gradient rises to several thousands
of volts per metre of height. Therefore, since a human being is usually
a little less than two metres tall, his head can be at a much higher potential than his lower parts. According to these differences in potential
we can classify the climates into four main types, three only of which
are mentioned and studied in biophysics:

1 Zones of strong climate. These are the regions where the atmospheric
electrical field is very high and where the voltage rises by at least 100
volts per metre. These zones correspond to what we call 'very invigorating health resorts'; they are physiologically stimulating.

2 Zones of average climate. Here the electrical potential difference varies
between 30 and 100 volts per metre. These health resorts are invigorating, but less stimulating than the zones of strong climate.

3 Zones of weak climate. Here the potential falls below 30 volts. These
regions have much lower vital activity than the two just mentioned
and they have a calming effect on very nervous people.

4 Zones of zero climate. Created by man, these are the inhabited areas
where he lives for about 300 days a year in the polluted atmosphere
of offices and apartments. Any person living in these zones, where the
potential is almost zero, should go and gather strength and revitalise
himself in zones of strong climate and recharge his nervous batteries.
    To choose a place for a holiday these different climates must be
recognised, and certain criteria will help. First the look of the country, then the type of vegetation, since the latter depends as much on
the climate as on the composition of the soil itself. After all, the soil
has been created as much by the plants themselves as by the mineral:
below:

(a) *Zones of strong climate*. These are almost always wide plateaux, or plains with broad horizons, where nothing stops the wind from blowing across them; the coasts of the North Sea and Atlantic are perfect examples. Vegetation is not luxuriant. Tall deciduous trees are absent. Conifers feel at home here, as they do in alpine regions too.

(b) *Zones of average climate*. These are more sheltered sites, near rocks or in valleys, close to woods and forests, in the plains and in deep coastal bays, sheltered from the sea wind. Vegetation here is far more abundant than in the zones of strong climate, without, however, being luxuriant. There are many deciduous trees, without being thickly wooded; there are pastures and poplars.

(c) *Zones of weak climate*. These include, amongst others, very deep valleys and areas of undergrowth, and the banks of deep-cut rivers. Here is vegetation particularly luxuriant, and rich in climbing plants. Ferns are abundant, so are evergreens. Thus, conifers without ferns indicate strong climates, conifers with ferns indicate weak climates. As to the fourth climate, no description is necessary.

Local variations. The regions described are not always of great area. In a region of very strong climate one finds a few restricted areas where the potential falls below one hundred or even below thirty volts, while on some North Sea beaches the potential may be even higher than one hundred volts, and fifty yards away, amongst the dunes, the potential may be that of a weak climate. In the hotel rooms, with the windows shut, it might be zero. Four climates may thus be found within the radius of a few hundred yards.

Our towns are unhealthy, not only because of the almost total absence of the active little negative ions (even in zones of strong climate houses several storeys high transform the streets into canyons of weak climate) but also because of the accumulation of car exhaust gases and the bacteria carried in the dust raised by the traffic. This information may help in the choice of the ideal setting and in avoiding the error of thinking that simply by living in a coastal town one will benefit automatically from the advantages of a strong climate.

Too rapid successions

Let us draw attention to yet another rule. Frail people must avoid a too rapid change of climate. During a bicycle ride through a wide valley we may pass through a zone of average climate; then the valley becomes narrower and we ride along wooded paths, that is to say in a zone of weak climate. We climb up the hill to admire the view and there we are in a zone of strong climate. Now only people in perfect health can run the risk of passing directly from one climate to another. Nature has given man two legs, which allow him to move about, even if at a relatively slow pace. But a car, which is in fact a moving electro- magnetic cage, luckily insulates man from the surrounding electric field and prevents him from suffering the consequences of abrupt climatic changes which he would encounter in the open air while travelling across the whole country in a single day.

If you observe your own reactions to these different types of climate you will discover some interesting facts and you will learn which climates suit you best. This is very important from every point of view; when we study cases of exceptional longevity and their geographical distribution we find that these occur particularly amongst people of the mountains. The Balkans are the region of centenarians and the oldest citizen of the USSR, who still rides a horse, has never left his native mountains. Independent of other factors, the Hunza people remain in their small territory in the Himalaya. It seems, moreover, that a balance establishes itself between the soil, the climate, the vegetation and the other living creatures, including man, in any given place. It is not desirable to disturb this balance frequently. Healthy peasants often lived fifty years and more on the same soil without ever leaving their villages.

On the other hand, it is certain that a radical but temporary change of climate can be favourable. It is good to go periodically to a zone of strong climate provided we stay there long enough for the organism to get used to it and for the pranic readjustment to take place. A change of climate is an 'aggression' which can be stimulating.

Thus, as we have seen, man is permanently under the influence of cosmic energy, which pours torrents of prana upon him. The sun is the nearest source of this and cosmic rays exercise an influence upon living beings which is still ill-defined but which is still very important. On the other hand, the earth, which absorbs and stores these energies, constitutes a second pole. The human organism, a vibrant electrical system, is the seat of incessant exchanges with the surrounding cosmic and terrestrial energies. Man has to avoid insulating himself behind screens, walls, windows, clothing and shoes. The lungs and slun are our exchange surfaces with the outer world; they are real electrical sponges, and we must lead the prana they absorb to our cells.

We must bear these ideas in mind in our daily conduct; it would be a serious mistake to ignore them. Pranayama gives us the psycho-physiological techniques necessary for the control and conscious use of these energies for our physical and psychic fulfilment.

4 | Prana in the Organism

'When we consider organic life in the light of biophysics, we find that electrical phenomena are at the root of all cellular life and we conclude that the end of everything is an electric charge.' (Dr J. Belot).

The study of bioelectric — or pranic — phenomena takes on a special importance when one visualises its practical applications, the purpose of which is to accumulate and 'manipulate' prana, for it is essential to understand why and how pranayama acts on our bodies through these subtle energies. For this purpose we shall quote from the works of several Western scientists which support yogic theories with the scientific rigour of the West and which enable us to understand the mechanism of Chinese acupuncture, an empirical form of medicine with an energising — or pranic — basis.

Preceding sections have shown that the yogic conception of prana has been confirmed by modern physics. We shall now turn our attention to an aspect of the problem which interests us particularly, namely the prana contained in the human body, and we shall see that here too yogic conceptions and advanced scientific thought meet.

Let us first consider the cell, the building brick of the human structure. For yogis, in the immense pranic ocean that constitutes the material universe, everything that lives, from the most humble cell to the most developed being, represents an organised whirlpool of energy. Prana is the basic energy that animates every form of life. Prana is not the so-called raw material but rather the energy that activates it. Prana accompanies life from its beginning, maintains and controls it. Each cell, considered individually, is the seat of important pranic manifestations (the yogis realised the existence of the cells, the 'little lives') and the entire organism is controlled by prana. Let us consider these points in detail.

Dr Rene Allendy writes:

'For a long time a certain scepticism, a reaction to the mysticism of bygone ages, an excessive tendency to a tangible objectivity, and a corrupted derivation of the true scientific spirit, have dissuaded doctors from the study of intangible things. And yet it is at the level of the infinitely small and the intangible that the vital mechanisms have their origin. This applies to normal phenomena as well as to the manifestation of disease, to pathological change as well as to the healing process. Many of these imponderables have already been accepted by science, and medical examinations should above all be conducted in that direction.

'For a long time, the cell has been considered as the first element of life and to relate all medical considerations to its level seemed the height of generalisation. This was the time of histology and of pathological anatomy. It seemed that nothing vital existed on a smaller scale. By contrast, today the cell appears to us to be an extremely complex organism.

'It appears that the vital mechanisms, particularly assimilation and elimination which together constitute nutrition, are linked to variations which are not only atomic but even electronic at the extremities of long chains in the organic molecule. An infinitely small modification of ions, atoms or electrons causes the fixation at this extremity of a new atom (absorption) or, on the contrary, the detachment of the chain (elimination). The molecule maintains itself in a state of relative equilibrium or of conservation by constant variations of this kind. "'We must study the disposition of the molecules and atoms, their nature and their electronic quantum levels in order to try to discover the principle of these processes, of this metabolism which is life." So writes Robert Tourmaire in his remarkable work *La Naissance de la Vie* (Paris, 1938, p. 136). In the past medicine and biology saw life as a simple chemical reaction, that is to say a completely mechanical exchange of atoms and molecules. Though this is still true, we can today interpret it more exactly for we now understand that these exchanges depend on an electric potential so that the essence of this phenomenon is moved from the atom to the electron. Thus, nutrition, like the gas exchanges in the lungs, is an electrical phenomenon. 'Professor Pech of Montpellier (Siècle Médical, June-November 1927) defined a nutrition index which was the difference of electrical potential between two tissues of a living being, or between the tissue of a living being and a substance, chemically defined or not, with which it is in contact, or between the tissue of a living being and the interior or exterior medium in relation to which it is nourished. This index is positive or negative relative to the tissue of the living being envisaged; sea water will have a negative index for man but artificially salinated water will have a positive index. Thus the problem of nutrition passes from chemistry to physics and becomes subject to the most subtle influences we know. Also flocculation of colloids, to which Auguste Lumière attributes the ageing process and a great many diseases, is due to the fact that the micelles lose their electric charges.'

To sum up we quote Dr Goust: 'Ionisation is of capital importance to the cells. The electrolytes have a biological activity caused by their ionisation. The ions are the true workers of cells and organic tissues in the organism.' Thus we can in a way consider each cell as a dynamo and the human body as a vast bioelectric system.

A first impression could lead us to believe that the nervous system alone is the seat of electrical manifestations; its fibres and physical organisation remind us of our telephone and electricity networks, while the brain appears as a computer charged with co-ordinating its functioning. Bioelectric phenomena control all the vital phenomena at all levels. It is true that pranic variations of electric potential, which take place along the nerves, form the nervous influx, but the circulation and transmission of bioenergy are not limited to the nervous system alone. Vlès has shown us that our organism is the seat of virtual electrical metabolism: the body absorbs cosmic energy and uses it internally for all the vital processes and then rejects a part of this energy by way of a constant loss of electrons. Wilhelm Reich has proved, with the help of measuring apparatus which he devised, that the transmission of bioenergy is not limited to the nervous system, but follows all the membranes .and fluids in the body. This hypothesis verifies the theory of Fr Kraus of Berlin, who found that the body was 'activated by electrical processes'. The body is formed of countless interfaces between membranes and electrolytical fluids of varying composition and density. According to a well-known physical law, electrical tensions are set up at the interfaces between conducting fluids and membranes. The differences of density and structure of the membranes are echoed in the tensions and interfaces and bring about differences of potential as a result. Thus our bodies are composed of countless internal surfaces with different energy potentials. The bioelectrical energy in our bodies is in constant movement, circulating from points of higher to points of lower potential in search of an equilibrium which is never reached. These electrical charges in continual search of equilibrium are carried by particles of body fluid, the ions,i.e. atoms bearing electrical charges. They are called 'cations' or 'anions' according to whether they move towards the negative or positive pole.

The special importance of this is that according to yogic theories the body is capable of storing energy and directing it at will. According to yogis our whole body is saturated with prana, so that it has to be thought of as an accumulator and transformer. Our vitality finally depends on a sufficient assimilation of prana and on its correct use. We shall now quote some Western sources that will enable us to set the yogic theories on a solid scientific basis. First, Dr Biancini:

'In biology electrical phenomena are of capital importance. Every act of nutrition and movement produces electricity. To the act of nutrition continuous so-called rest currents correspond; the functioning of the organs is linked to intermittent currents called action currents.

'The rest currents arise from the chemical action taking place in the protoplasm. Thus living tissue can be compared to an infinity of minute batteries.

'The action currents, which we can demonstrate at the level of the muscles, nerves, glands and skin, can be explained by the relation which links electrical phenomena and capillary actions. The variations of electrical potential cause variations of surface tension and the phenomena of osmosis determine the variations of electrical potential.

'Variations of surface tension and mechanical deformation occur constantly in living tissues, hence the constant production of electricity. These facts explain that in an organism the potential differences are linked to the vital processes. The less active regions are electro-negative compared with the more vital regions.

'Some years ago, together with the late Dr Dimier, a renowned electrologist, we carried out some investigations into the existence and extent of human electricity. A highly sensitive galvanometer enabled us to perceive this electricity and we found that the Chinese acupuncture points had a particularly strong transmitting power. It was even possible, by linking with a copper wire the two San-li points on the legs of the same person, and by amplifying the wave, to note the presence of a continuous current between the two sides of the body. Numerous observations were made which showed that with persons in good health the electrical charge averaged eight micro-amperes; the figure for tired people was barely one or two micro-amperes, while for over excited or tense people it rose to fifteen.

'It is fair to suppose that what we call "life force" is above all this electrical potential, and that when we feel weary and say "my batteries are flat" the expression can be taken almost literally. Without seeking to reduce them to electricity, vitality and health show their presence by an abundant bioelectrical charge, by ion exchanges and by the tension of the electrical potential and the harmony of all functions. That is to say, good health depends more on the distribution and harmonious diffusion of these "currents" than is generally believed. The figure of fifteen micro-amperes found in over excited persons shows that they really live in a state of perpetual "short-circuit", "bursting their batteries" .'

Reich has written as follows, a passage which we would do well to ponder upon:

'A new approach to the understanding of organic disease opens before us. We now look at neuroses in a totally different way from the psychoanalists. They are not only the result of unresolved psychic conflicts or childhood fixations. Rather, these fixations and conflicts cause fundamental disturbances of the bioelectrical system and so get anchored somatically. That is why we think it is impossible to separate the psychic from the somatic processes.' It follows that if a man were able to store this bioelectrical energy and direct and distribute it at will within his body he would possess the key to physical and mental health. This is the first objective of pranayama.

What we have been discussing helps us to understand how Chinese acupuncture works. If we had not discovered this production, ingestion and circulation of electrical energy in the fluids and tissues of the human body, as well as its organisation in currents, the process of acupuncture would have remained incomprehensible.

Soulie de Morant has written:

'According to several electrologists the acupuncture needles cause an electrical discharge from the body into the air. I have often been able to verify that an amplifier on a silver needle implanted in an appropriate point in a contracted muscle will pick up the rapid vibrations of a wave. In some cases this could also be detected by the finger and a discharge would be felt to travel along the hand and the arm, thereby numbing them.

'Currents flow continuously between our negatively charged bodies and the usually positively charged air. Their action is uncertain, but they seem to control the stimulation of the peripheral and central nervous systems and thereby of the whole organism. At any given point the atmospheric electrical potential undergoes continuous and often large variations (sometimes up to 30 per cent) even in fine weather and when there is no apparent reason. These accidental variations, which are particularly noticeable in daytime, differ considerably from one point to another, even when close. In bad weather (storm, clouds, rain, fog or snow) the variations may even reach from 3,000 to 5,000 volts and in less than a minute change from thousands of positive volts to negative values of the same order. A strong wind reduces the potential sometimes to the extent of changing its polarity."

'Tonification and dispersal are words with no precise meaning for most Europeans but they are very clear to anyone who understands energetics. Tonification is the transfer of energy to a part of the organism from another part which is its yin-yang opposite. As the energy drives and stimulates the blood, this generally causes an increase in circulation, in the nourishment of the organs and an increase in vitality. Dispersal is the scattering of energy concentrated in one part of the organism over parts of the body which are its yin-yang opposites, thereby reducing the excess of vitality and circulation, relieving congestion and pain.

'The methods used for tonification and dispersal also depend on yin-yang. A passage in the Nei Tsing of the twenty-eight century BC tells how before the discovery of copper and fine needles it had been noticed that wounds caused a loss of colour and depressed the system while burns stimulated warmth and life. This led to the invention for the purpose of dispersal first of stone spikes and then of fine copper needles, and for the purpose of tonification first of fire-brands and then of *tsiou* , which we call "moxas" (from the Japanese *mogusa* , a burning herb), a word that has come down to us through the Dutch. At that time the needles were supposed capable only of causing dispersal, whilst the moxas were always used for tonification in preference to needles.

'Fairly quickly, however, observations led the Chinese to discover that pricks and burns on certain points of the body not only had a general effect but also had repercussions on one or other organ. Later still, but doubtless before the twenty-eighth century BC, it was found that certain points always had a tonifying whereas other points had a dispersing action. From this time onwards almost all the points were known. It was then that the "meridians" were discovered, the lines on which the points are situated, each organ having its series of resonating and excitation points and its meridian. At the same time it was discovered that these meridians communicated with each other by their extremities. Lastly, many patients had stated that they felt "a certain something" all along the meridian at the moment of pricking. This "certain something" always went in the same direction in the meridian which was being treated and from there passed to the meridian linked with it. The circulation of energy which stimulates alternatively the yin and the yang had been discovered.

'The meridians of this circulation of energy follow no other known vector such as nerves or arteries, etc. The Chinese consider that this circulation is in communication through the high point, *Trong-t'ien*, with the cosmic energy, Yang, and through the low point, *Trae-tsri*, with the earth's energy, Yin. The organism would thus be like an accumulator-transformer of yin-yang.'

5 | Prana and the Astronauts

In teaching yoga and its techniques I make every effort to invent nothing and to follow as closely as possible the spirit and letter of yoga, going to the most authentic sources (to which, fortunately, I have access) and adding the product of my own experience through more than twenty-five years. My contribution lies principally in the realm of the 'cuisine': yoga supplies me with the raw materials which I accommodate to the tastes and needs of the Western world to make them palatable. That is all.

One of my personal contributions is that I seem to have been the first to establish a correlation between certain scientific discoveries and the yogic theory of prana. Relying on Western research that has been carried out without any connection to yoga, I am convinced that one of the forms, if not the main form, of the prana of the air is constituted by the free negative ions, tiny packets of electrical energy borne by the oxygen atoms of the air, and that this energy is assimilated by our organisms.* One author has stated his belief that prana is the same as ozone or even the rare gases (neon, argon, etc.), an opinion which I do not share. These gases, like oxygen or nitrogen, are chemical constituents of the air, whereas the yogic texts are very definite: prana is the subtle energy 'of the same nature as lightning' but distinct from air itself. I shall complete here what I have said previously, as this is a fundamental aspect of pranayama and even of yoga as a whole.

The following pages will show how far the brilliant intuition of the Rishis and sages of old India is confirmed by Western science and they will show the tremendous importance of prana in human biology. I am convinced that medical treatment in the future will be pranic!

First I quote an article which appeared in *Le Monde* of 24–25 March 1968 on the 'Medical and Scientific News' page. It was entitled 'The influence of atmospheric electricity on health as studied by specialists at Briançon':

'Briançon - March. The health resort of Briançon was host to a

---

* I have published articles on this subject in the monthly journal Yoga, which I have edited since 1965.

one-day congress on atmospheric ionisation organised by the Briançon centre for bioclimatic research. From this congress it became evident that much research is needed in the field of atmospheric electricity. The contributions, which were sometimes contradictory, showed the need for close collaboration between doctors and physicists. The need for diversity of approach, for methodology of research, and for serious centralised information also became apparent. This would avoid work being carried out in isolation in this field, which deals with the qualitative and quantitative repercussions on living beings of electrically charged particles in the atmosphere.

'The work done in the underwater research laboratory in Toulon, and presented by Dr Vogt, interested participants at the congress, which was chaired by Professor Bricart of the University of Paris. The experiments of the Toulon laboratory deal mainly with the effects of atmospheric ions in excess. From this study it appears that the action of negative ions causes a modification of respiratory constants (increase in partial pressure of oxygen in the air cells of the lungs and decrease in that of carbon dioxide) while positive ions have the reverse effect.'

The last paragraph is crucial: it shows that in the lungs the presence of negative ions favours the passage of oxygen through the air cell membranes so that this oxygen is more efficiently absorbed by the blood. At the same time, the removal of carbon dioxide is also made easier. The overall result is an increased oxygen fixation and easier and more complete rejection of carbon dioxide. The article continues:

'Furthermore, the excess of positive ions causes a reduction in the vital respiratory capacity and in the maximum expired volume. It does not seem to cause a marked change in the circulatory system although other tests suggest that positive ions may cause a deterioration in psycho-physiological performance.'

In earlier pages on atmospheric prana we have said that industry emits thousands of tons of dust of which each particle is a trap for the vitalising negative ions. This causes a catastrophic reduction of free negative ions and an alarming increase in harmful positive ions. This conclusion throws unexpected light on the problem of atmospheric pollution. We think of the pollution of towns as being mainly due to poisonous gases and residues (carbon monoxide, sulphur dioxide, and nitric oxide emitted by factories, heating installations and motor cars) while dust is often thought to be harmless. No doubt these toxic gases attack the respiratory tracts and poison the organism, but the almost complete suppression of negative ions by dust and the increase in positive ions which reduce our vitality attack us insidiously through out vital forces. Our eliminating organs (kidneys, liver, etc.) can to a certain extent neutralise and eliminate these poisons with the exception of carbon monoxide, which irreversibly blocks the haemoglobin. On the other hand, *nothing* compensates for the loss of vitality of which town dwellers, forced to breathe air without prana, are the victims. This reduction in vitality saps our natural immunity to pathogenic germs, which according to Claude Bernard only become virulent in a weakened host. The fight against pollution should, therefore, treat dust in the same way as any other pollutant.

Air-conditioning
We Westerners are proud of the fact that we have 'improved' the air we breathe. Specialists have measured its temperature, humidity and so on, and many buildings have been fitted at great expense with air-conditioning equipment designed to give 'ideal' standard air, the last word in comfort and hygiene. However, the 'privileged' persons who benefit – often against their will – from these installations seem far less enthusiastic than the inventors (and the sellers) of air-conditioning plant. Those condemned to work in air-conditioned offices often regret having left the old building: they say, 'At least we could open the windows.' This can be explained by the prana in the air. After passing through the air-conditioner where all the negative ions have been caught, the air has become inert, devoid of any vitalising power. People who have to breathe this air feel exhausted after the day's work: they often suffer from migraine, have a reduced work output and a reduced power of concentration. The air has become unbearable and people who breathe it live on their reserves, using the few other sources of prana (e.g. food) which are themselves of reduced value. Today's air-conditioning is indeed conditioning in reverse. But who listens to such arguments, even today? Gradually, however, the truth penetrates. We read:

'Artificial ionisation and air-conditioning
'Andre Langevin, an engineer from the University of Paris, discussed

the problem of air-conditioning. An air-conditioning plant which gives a constant temperature and a humidity of between 40 and 70 per cent and which removes dust from new air must today be considered incomplete. In order to complete such a plant, Langevin considers it necessary to include a method of producing artificial atmospheric ions.

'Other important work has shown that ions participate in all vital functions: it would be particularly desirable to study in more detail the way the negative oxygen ions act on the organism in order to ascertain whether these ions act as catalysts for the oxygenation of the blood.

'In the meantime, according to Langevin, it would be useful to tell users of air-conditioning not to neglect the need for some ionisation, a factor which so far has been almost completely ignored. Artificial ionisation should improve the abnormal living conditions of most town dwellers.'

These lines thus condemn all existing air-conditioning plants. It could be argued that the removal of dust by air-conditioners is an important positive factor. It is certainly important to have dust-free air, but the dust should be stopped at the source, by trapping it at the factory which emits it. Once in the atmosphere, it is too late, the damage has been done. These ion traps must be prevented from devitalising the air we breathe. The only way to do this is to stop them from entering the air; anything else is illusory.

The preceding paragraphs also confirm 'that ions participate in all vital functions', a sentence which should be published in millions of copies to haunt those responsible. 'Negative ions take part in all vital functions.' They are catalysts for the oxygenation of the blood. Those who remove these negative ions interfere with all vital functions and consequently with the health of entire populations.

Langevin mentions artificial ionisation which is being seriously studied in several countries. This research began as part of the application of biophysics to interplanetary journeys in the space programme. The astronauts are chosen with the utmost care; they are a physical, psychological and mental elite. They must be robust and in perfect health, able to resist the trials of launching, orbital flight and return to earth in a space capsule. They must also have the courage and psychic energy necessary to overcome the nervous stress created by waiting in the capsule for the moment of launching, by the feeling of being cut off from the world and by the cramped conditions. Furthermore, the astronaut is required to be simultaneously a physicist, mathematician, astronomer, engineer, mechanic and who knows what else, as he can count only on himself to maintain his equipment during the long interplanetary journeys which are already under consideration. It has been observed that these specially chosen men, well trained and well nourished, nevertheless become tired unusually quickly in their space capsules; their concentration diminishes, their excellent reflexes become slower and less precise, and they complain of a vague feeling of exhaustion. This could be attributed to weightlessness but for the fact that the same symptoms occur during training sessions on the ground.

No biophysicist would have thought of asking the advice of a yogi, who could have put his finger on the root of the problem at once. 'There is no prana in this capsule,' he would have said, 'and thus the human being is no longer linked to the big cosmic dynamo, the inexhaustible reservoir of universal prana. He lives on his reserves and as these are not progressively reconstituted they are, of course, very quickly exhausted.'

However, research was quickly directed towards the electrical properties of the air and now there are machines which enable man to recreate the electromagnetic conditions of the free air. This research was labelled 'top secret' for a long time and in the USA was catalogued under 'Title 35 Code US – 1952, Sections 181– 188'. Today it is no longer secret, for it has become apparent that the Russian 'competitors' had encountered the same problem and seem to have solved it. The following information came from the American firm which produces these negative ion generators: 'It has been established beyond doubt that an electric field exists between the earth and the atmosphere. This natural electric field is normally positive (in relation to the earth) and its strength is usually of the order of several hundred volts per metre.'

We may refer the reader to Section 3 in which we dealt with the potential gradient. In order to simplify matters we made no mention of the idea of the electric field. We concentrated on the negative ions. What part does the positive field play? The negative ions fly about at high altitude, where they are produced mainly by the ionising effect of solar radiation. They would stay there indefinitely as the earth is charged negatively, except for the fact that near to the ground there exists a positive electrical field. We must not confuse the 'electric field' with the 'ions'. Because it has direction the field is a vectoral quantity;

it is not materialised in the form of ions. The ions are the carriers of electric energy whereas the electric field acts as a force which moves these ions either by attraction or by repulsion according to circumstances. The ions behave like iron filings attracted by a magnetic field. Thus the flow of negative ions comes down to earth only if a positive electric field attracts them. With this made clear we are better able to understand the rest of the text: 'In living quarters which are insulated and which have the properties of a Faraday cage, there is no electric field.' This is what I meant when I said that in certain apartments the potential gradient is zero.

'…The electric field of the earth is a natural electric force which produces beneficial effects on living organisms and to which man has become adapted over several thousands of years. Indeed, evolution has without doubt taken account of this factor. Experiments have shown that the electric field produces an electric current inside the body which stimulates the whole organism and its nervous system which, in turn, increases the activity of the brain…'

But we soon meet again the negative ions with which we are familiar.

'The beneficial effects attributed to the electric field are due to the combined action of the positive electric field and the negative ions which are freely suspended in the atmosphere. The electric field is the cause of the movement but the ions carry the electric charge. A continuous electric current passes through the atmosphere and the whole human body. Under normal atmospheric conditions this continuous electric current is of the order of 10–12 amps through the body taken as a whole, i.e. approximately 10–16 amp seconds per cm^2.'

These currents are very weak but that does not prevent them from being of vital importance. At the level of a drop of water the attraction of the moon is an absolutely negligible force. At the scale of oceans it causes one of the most important cosmic phenomena on the surface of the globe. '

As there are always ions in free suspension in the air [note: the quantity varies enormously and in certain cases there are almost no favourable negative ions] it is the presence of the positive electric field and its intensity which are the most important factors in the creation of this continuous electric current through the human body and which are therefore at the root of the beneficial physiological effects…

'…The electric current caused by the presence of an electric field passes through all the cells, the organs and the whole of the nervous system, and stimulates the metabolism as well as all other physiological functions of living organisms.

'… If the organism remains in a room or space where there is no positive electric field (as in a Faraday cage) or even if the field is too weak, tiredness, indolence, and lack of vitality will be manifest. This is the main cause of tiredness and numbness felt in cars, planes, tanks, submarines, and trains and now also in space capsules. In all these cases experience indicates that the creation of a controlled artificial electric field is probably the only efficient, infallible and completely safe means of retarding considerably the onset of tiredness, exhaustion and sleepiness. The physiological effects of artificial electric fields are identical to those of the natural electric field…'

We emphasise that it is above all the very special conditions of a space capsule which have shown the importance of this factor. The report quoted states:

'Being wholly metallic, each space capsule is an absolutely ideal Faraday cage in which even the best trained space pilot quickly shows signs of physiological disturbances (for example in his cardio-vascular functioning, in his metabolism, in his electrolytic equilibrium, etc.) and particularly tiredness and early exhaustion. These physiological disturbances have been noted without doubt during American orbital flights. They have been observed in a similar competent manner and openly admitted by the Russians. Glenn as well as Carpenter tired very quickly, and tiredness as well as exhaustion and physiological disturbance were such in the case of the space pilot Titov that he was actually air-sick after only six orbits. These embarrassing phenomena, which showed themselves right from the beginning of space exploration, were seriously dscussed during the Symposium held at the space centre, Houston, 21 September 1962.

Surprisingly, however, the two Russian pilots Nikolayev and Popovitch showed no sign of tiredness during their twin flights in August 1962, although these had lasted 96 and 72 hours respectively. The two pilots showed unusual vitality. To try to explain this extraordinary vitality by their previous training would be an error. It is even less likely that the special vitality of the two Russian pilots was due to the taking of drugs. The only possible explanation for this is to admit that even at that time the Russians were already using successfully the same techniques as that of the American machine called an anti-fatigue unit.'

Research was carried out in the USA with great scientific precision; I shall not go into the details here, as it is only the facts and results that interest us. Research was also carried out on the influence of electric (read 'pranic') currents in medicine.

'Dr Daniel established that attacks of prolonged coughing diminished quite spectacularly in patients treated by an electric field. This can be understood electrophysiologically in the light of the latest research concerning the conversion of the inhaled oxygen fixed by the body cells which transform it, especially the heart cells.

'The importance of this principle and its application to vast fields become evident when we consider the latest discoveries of Professor Wartburg of Germany regarding cancer cells. When healthy cells are put into a position where it becomes impossible for them to breathe normally, they pass into a state of "fermentation" and then become true cancer cells.

'The energy necessary for assimilation by digestion is obtained through the intermediary of the air of the atmosphere by means of an extremely complex electrical process. During this process adenosine triphosphate acid, which is particularly rich in energy, seems to be the carrier of this energy. In nature the electrostatic field exercises an important influence on the "respiration-phosphorisation" chain during which the oxygen of the air becomes "active" to a corresponding degree.

'Consequently the application of electrostatic fields has become part of the treatment for cardiac occlusions (infarctus) or angina pectoris. All the patients of Dr Daniel who received this treatment have undeniably benefited from it.'

Some conclusions

The same authors note the repercussions which result from an absence of electric fields and currents:

'The absence of an electric current is *always* a disadvantage and *always* has negative effects on the vitality of the human being and can even dangerously influence his fertility: – the longevity of civilised man depends to a very high degree on the continual presence of a sufficiently powerful electric field;
– the most important physiological functions – cardiac activity, respiration, digestion, metabolism, etc. – are favourably influenced and stimulated by this electric field;
– a great many so-called "modern illnesses" can be traced to the absence or considerable reduction in intensity of the natural electrical fields in big towns;
– human beings who are forced to live in buildings or rooms with metal frames and which therefore have the physical properties of a Faraday cage, from which any electric field is excluded, tire and are exhausted quickly .'

It is fortunate that the absence of prana influences the productivity of the human being, for in our consumer society health is of less importance than productivity. Anything that reduces productivity becomes *ipso facto* important. It is therefore probable that in the name of productivity research will be carried out and the appropriate measure taken to preserve or reconstitute the natural electric (pranic) field whenever necessary.

Negative electric fields

We have seen that in nature the element which is charged with the active electric energy, the negative ion, is drawn towards earth by a positive electric field which exists at ground level and in the lower layers of the atmosphere. Thus we have a continuous downward current between the upper layers of the atmosphere, which are negatively ionised, and the positive electric field in which the human being lives and moves when he is in the open. We have seen the disastrous consequences of the suppression of this electric field and the capture of the negative ions by dust, smoke, etc., which are suspended in the atmosphere particularly above large industrial cities. Now let us examine what happens when the charges are reversed, that is to say when the electric field becomes negative and the ions positive.

In the journal *Product Engineering* of 13 February 1967, published in the USA, we read:

'Negative fields: certain spaces formed of plastic like car bodies can even produce negative electric fields (fields which reject negative ions and attract positive ions). Plastic furniture as well as plastic seat and wall coverings accelerate mental fatigue in the occupants of the room or the vehicle.

'Objects and coverings in polyethylene, for example, produce negative electric fields from 5,000 to 10,000 voltslmetre: in a space completely enclosed by polyethylene the negative field may reach 100,000 volts / metre.'

This proves that we must be very careful even in the choice of materials which surround us and in our clothing. Who has not worn underclothes (men's shirts, and so on) which stick to the skin and are attracted by the body when taken off? Sometimes even sparks fly and the hairs on the skin stand up as we take off a shirt. In another article, published in January 1964 in *Aerospace Medicine* we find these words:

'Clothes are important for the same reason. Certain synthetic materials produce enough electrostatic negative charges to repel the negative ions from the person wearing the clothing...'

Thus, even if we are in a correctly ionised environment, clothes can partially nullify the beneficial effect of the negative health-giving ion stream. Luckily we can capture prana with the mucous membranes of the nose and absorb it directly. Cotton clothing is recommended as it does not modify the electric field or the ionic currents. We should live as much as possible in the open air, far from towns, in order to top up our pranic batteries. Condemned as we are to passing a good deal of our existence under unfavourable pranic conditions, yogic methods for the fixing of prana are all the more useful.

6 | Prana-absorbing Organs

'The first aim of yoga is the control of vital energies or prana (so called since the vital breath, prana, is the most important and the most directly controllable of all vital rhythms). To this end we must first establish control by our mental consciousness of all our vital and emotional reactions. This absorption by the conscious self of inframental energies gives us the strength which enables the conscious self to penetrate the regions of supramental conscience...

'The name Hatha Yoga has been given to the practices and disciplines which enable us to control our bodies and energies. Though this is only one of the means of yoga, it is the first preparation on the road to reintegration, the necessary starting point for a further realisation.' (Alain Danielou, *Methode de reintegration*)

In the preceding sections we have called upon the evidence of modern science for an explanation of pranic theory, but in fact prana and the techniques of pranayama do not need its support. For the yogis the essential thing is that the system works and produces the expected results. In this field they have at least four or five thousand years' experience and are that much ahead of us! Yet it is reassuring for the modern reader to find that as far as prana is concerned Western science has confirmed the yogis' theories.

What exactly does 'pranayama' mean? The word is composed of 'prana' and 'ayama', the latter meaning length, expansion, retention and also control. Pranayama is thus the yogic science of the control of prana in the human being. It will be observed that we did not write 'human body', for pranayama covers more than the physical aspect. Pranayama is the most vital of sciences since ultimately all energies which show themselves in the form of life are pranic: every human being from life to death handles prana without, however, being involved in pranayama. The aim of yoga is to intensify and consciously control this pranic metabolism in order to multiply the physical, mental and psychic energies of the adept. To regard pranayama simply as breathing exercises or breath control is to give too narrow a view, for breath control is not the aim – it is only the means, albeit a very efficient one, of learning to control and distribute the vital energies.

Our organisms are in constant communication with the cosmos, impregnated as it is with pranic energy vibrations. The essential difference between an inanimate object – whether a chair or the most perfected robot – and a living being, from amoeba to man, is that the former is passively subject to the action of cosmic forces, whereas the latter takes the prana, transforms it and uses it for its own ends. We exist by constantly drawing prana from the cosmos and this extraction takes place by means of specialised organs. For the yogis the main points of prana absorption are as follows, in order of importance: (1) the nerve endings in the nasal cavities, (2) the air-cells in the lungs, (3) the tongue, (4) the skin. We shall now study them one by one, starting with that of least importance for prana control.

The skin
The skin is more than a mere envelope: it is one of the largest and most important organs of the body. Without it we cannot survive, as has been proved in cases of severe burning. Its function as an eliminating organ is well known to the public, but not its role in absorbing vitality. Through the pores we eliminate toxic substances which would otherwise accumulate in the body; what is much less well known and what interests us particularly is the pranic role of the skin. It is – or should be – in contact with the air which is vibrant with energy, for it can absorb directly large quantities of solar prana, according to yogic theory. This places sunbathing in a fresh light, for with the yogis it goes far beyond the simple objective of acquiring a suntan, all the more so in India where the ambition to be sunburnt does not exist; on the contrary, a light skin is what most people admire. For the yogis, exposing the skin to the sun means absorbing the radiant solar energy. In the West we believe that the skin reacts automatically to the action of the sun's rays; which is true, but the yogis believe that it is possible to influence this absorption of energy, to increase it and to control it. Although the main role of the skin is to absorb prana, it also serves to eliminate it. In previous sections we have learned that the skin is an important emitter of electrical energy.

Knowledge of the laws of prana control, dealt with later, will permit us to sunbathe actively in order to use the time of exposure to the best advantage, very important because those opportunities do not occur frequently. When shall we have clothing which will protect us from inclement weather without insulating us from cosmic prana? Meanwhile we must let sun and air reach our skin whenever possible.

The tongue

'You are what you eat.' We are condensed sunlight. This grain of wheat, this salad leaf and this apple, are they not concentrated solar energy?

To the yogis the tongue is an important organ of prana absorption. A considerable part of the body's energy is extracted from food, and to a Westerner it seems to be our only source of energy, our real 'fuel'. And if we regard the body merely as a thermal engine without further examination the view is justifiable and we do not, in any case, deny the importance of diet (see *Yoga Self-taught*). However, this applies only to the solid aspect of the body, for as soon as we enter the realm of the subtle, vital energies, pranic by definition, these physical constituents become less important. From the pranic point of view, prana is absorbed not so much by the stomach and intestines as by the tongue.

The yogis link prana with taste: so long as a food has flavour it still contains some prana which can be extracted. (To be clear, flavour is not prana, it only indicates its presence.) The yogis continue to chew their food until it becomes tasteless; at this point, after the subtle prana has been absorbed, they swallow it and the digestive system can transform and use it as building material for the body. The importance of chewing is thus seen in a very different light from the usual one – as a means to fascilitate digestion. If we do not chew our food until the flavour has been exhausted – since, according to yoga, no other prana-absorbing organs exist in the digestive tract – the food can certainly build the physical body but cannot top up our pranic batteries and supply energy. On reflection we must agree with the yogic theories. When we are worn out and tired we are quickly restored by eating; we get the impression that our dynamism has been revived and that we are ready to resume the yoke. But physiologically speaking the invigorating effect of a meal could only be felt, at the earliest, two or three hours later, not before digestion has begun. On the contrary, before food can produce energy, energy is used up: digestion, a very complex process, uses up 70 per cent of the available nervous energy. The yogic theory explains all this if it is realised that the pranic energy of food is absorbed by the tongue without digestion. Here we should remember that in homoeopathy the patient is advised to keep the medicament under his tongue for a long while; homoeopathic medicine may be more pranic than chemical, perhaps almost exclusively so.

The nose
Whatever importance we attach to the skin and the tongue, the yogis regard the nose as the main prana-absorbing organ. Our main nutrient is air; without it we pass from life to death within minutes and its insufficiency causes severe physiological troubles. At the rate of eighteen inhalations of one litre of air per minute on average, the nose enables about 13,000 litres to pass in every twenty-four hours. Compared with this, two litres of water and one kilo of solid food seem paltry.

As air is our main nutrient its passage is strictly monitored, so the nasal cavities are filled with an infinite number of ultra-sensitive nervous receptors which detect all qualitative variations of the air. The nose does no more than condition the air, freeing it from dust, warming and moistening it; but it also measures its subtle qualities. A bad smell immediately starts an important physiological mechanism: the body becomes alert because a bad smell could signify poison. The sensitivity of the nasal nervous receptors is incredible. Think for a moment of what happens when you catch the scent of a rose. The quantity of matter which emerges from the flower is so minute, so diluted – almost atomised – that only the highly perfected measuring instruments of nuclear physics can detect and measure it; yet the olfactory apparatus reacts immediately, not merely noting the scent but identifying it with precision – we recognise the scent of a rose at once, or a lily of the valley or a hyacinth. Humanity has always attached great importance to perfumes and has known from antiquity now to extract the essences, ionised and ionisable, of plants and flowers. Natural scents are carriers of prana, of bioelectricity.

Scent is an important and exciting element in the life of a plant. Its role is twofold: it attracts flying insects which gather nectar and ensure fertilisation, but it also acts negatively by repelling or even destroying certain micro organisms and parasites, even at a great distance. A pleasant smell encourages us to breathe deeply, probably because our bodies 'know' that it is good; to inhale the fragrance of flowers is to commune with nature as anyone who has smelt the Corsican maquis will understand.

Aromatherapy, the treatment of certain illnesses by inhaling balm, is coming back into fashion. It is, in a way, a sort of super-homoeo-opathy. Moreover, if I remember rightly, Hahnemann, the founder of homoeopathy, used greater and greater dilutions at the end of his life, and even reached the stage of allowing his patients merely to sniff the substance. Only natural fragrances work; synthetic products have no effect. According to the advocates of aromatherapy, the natural plant essence distributes its qualities rapidly throughout the organism, thanks to its 'subtlety' and its 'electric life', to use the terms employed by the defenders of this form of therapy.

'Carried by the blood stream, the ionised plant aroma impreg-nates every corner of the body, powerfully vitalises the polarised and discharged cells, replenishes electronic shortages by recharging the bioelectromagnetic batteries, and disperses the cellular residue by dis-solving the viscous and diseased substances of body fluids. It oxidises the poisonous metabolic waste products, increases the energy balance, frees the mechanism of organic oxidation and of self-regulation, and reaches the lungs and kidneys whence it is exhaled or excreted without trace. The powerful electrolytic charges of the aroma, by cleansing the cells, restart the waves of vibration by induction and re-establish the electro-sanguine exchanges within and between the tissues.' (Dr J. Valnet, L'Hôpital, Paris, 1961)

By definition, aromatherapy is based on the absorption by the nasal mucous membranes of volatile elements, ionised and made pranic. Moreover, by acting on the nerve endings in the nostrils, which are connected by reflex action to the nervous centres in the spinal cord, particularly in the medula oblongata, it is possible to produce deep and immediate reactions in all body functions.

A familiar example is our natural reaction when someone faints. We look at once for a bottle of smelling salts and make the victim inhale. In fact a person who has fainted is barely breathing; the ir-ritant gas is not felt in the lungs, which only an infinitesimal fraction reaches, but the gas acts upon the nerve endings in the nostrils and the victim soon breathes again, the heart beats faster and colour returns to the face, the eyes open and the fainter, astonished, asks what has happened. This shows to what extent the nostrils are connected with the vital nerve centres.[*]

Here we must mention nasal reflex therapy, a technique which raised great hopes, which have not been realised because of practical difficulties. By tickling certain precise spots in the nasal cavities one causes, by way of a reflex, reactions in distant organs, such as the stomach, liver, kidneys, spleen, etc. The therapeutic use of this phenomenon gave birth to nasal reflex therapy, but a major difficulty is that the zone which corresponds to a particular organ is of course minute and varies with every individual; the nervous geography of the nostrils is unique like a fingerprint. Extensive and patient individual research is necessary in each case in order to draw up a nasal 'map' before starting treatment. Furthermore, this therapy applies only in cases of recent functional disturbances and not to old troubles in the form of organic lesions. For these reasons the method has had to be abandoned, but it has confirmed that the nostrils are in reflex contact with the whole nervous mechanism controlling our bodily functions. These conclusions are very important as they enable us to understand the laws of accumulation of pranic energy as defined by the yogis.

The air cells (alveoli) of the lungs
The nostrils are the main organs of prana absorption, but the lungs, too, are the seat of important pranic activities. The passage of oxygen from alveoli into the blood depends very much on the physical (i.e. bioelectric) qualities of the blood.

Prana obeys thought
One of the most remarkable discoveries of the yogis, which alone would justify the study and practice of yoga, is that prana obeys thought. To put it another way, concentrated thought allows us to absorb a larger amount of prana. In this connection Hatha yoga, of which the practice of pranayama is the backbone – with asanas and relaxation – combines with Raja yoga, the yoga for the control of the mind, since the mind can consciously direct the absorption, storage and distribution of prana in the human body. Remember that the absorption and accumulation of prana are controlled by thought, for thought directs the practice of pranayama.

---

[*] The reader is referred to Section 24, pp. 144 ff.

7 | Taking the Air

Like sayings and proverbs, many ordinary expressions contain unexpected wisdom. Thus, when we say we are 'taking the air', we mean only that we are going outdoors to breathe the pure air as opposed to the confined indoor air. But the expression should be taken literally: we should really *take* the air instead of merely breathing it in almost passively as is generally the case with 'homo domesticus'. We are sedentary, civilised beings, and even in the pure air of the countryside, while breathing or trying to breathe in the yogic way – that is to say doing complete breathing – we certainly *inhale* the air but we do not *take* it.

What is the difference? For the wild animal living in nature and for primative man the air is an indispensable element of life – as it is for us – but in addition it carries an infinite amount of information. In fact, compared with animals, our sense of smell is atrophied. For animals the air carries a whole world of sensations and messages. It vibrates with emanations: the smell of an enemy on the alert or of prey hiding in the long grass of the swamp. Game hunters in Africa and Asia know very well that the wind carries their scent to the game and so gives a warning. They therefore take the direction of the wind into account when approaching their victims. Our own sense of smell is hardly used, except to appreciate the smells from the kitchen or artificial perfumes and, rarely, the scent of flowers.

When inhaling, an animal takes possession of the air through its often very mobile nostrils. Watch those of a rhinoceros in the zoo or of a rabbit in its hutch: they catch the air actively. Some tribes (e.g. in Africa) that have remained close to nature show that man in his 'natural' state also *catches* and *examines* the air with his nostrils. The nostrils are equipped with small muscles which in our case are inactive but which in the so-called 'savages' are very mobile, for each time they inhale their nostrils dilate to facilitate a true *acquisition* of air.

Try breathing this way. First breath normally – either ordinary breathing or the complete yogic breathing. The nostrils scarcely move. Then inhale deeply and energetically, while relaxing the nostrils, and observe that the suction caused by inhalation tends to draw them inwards, thus reducing the passage offered to the incoming air. It can even happen that one nostril becomes completely closed because of this suction.

Now try to 'take' the air. Inhale, while stiffening the nostrils' muscles (when exhaling we shall have to relax them). A few breaths taken in this manner will show that the air enters more easily, in greater volume and in a more balanced way (i.e. through *both* nostrils which, from the viewpoint of prana absorption, is extremely important.[*]) Opening the nostrils during inhalation not only facilitates the entry of more air but actively directs it upwards towards the area with the most sensitive nerve endings. While atrophied in comparison with those of animals living in a world of varied smells, our nasal nerve endings, whose work is to analyse and identify smells, are nonetheless remarkably sensitive.

Our noses are real pranic antennae. Dilation of the nostrils modifies the shape of the funnel formed by the lower part of the nose and guides the inhaled air towards those parts of the nasal cavities where the nerve endings are most numerous – the site, according to the yogis, of our principal pranic receiver.

It seems that this special arrangement of the nostrils triggers off by reflex mechanism a step-by-step change in the whole respiratory system. Beginning at the nostrils this may go as far as the bronchial tubes. It is possible that its influence may even reach the alveoli. The respiratory system, which is intimately linked with the nervous system, forms in many respects an organic whole. Just as biting into a fruit causes a flow of saliva and triggers off reactions in the entire digestive tract, even at points which the food has not yet reached,[**] so the active intake of air triggers off nervous mechanisms which influence the absorption of air at all levels of the respiratory system. Similarly, a nauseating smell immediately blocks the respiratory mechanism.

Lacking recent and precise scientific information on these chain reactions starting in the nasal cavities, we can nevertheless give a familiar example to support our statement: sneezing. A minor irritation of the nerve endings in the nasal cavities by reflex action causes a violent response in the entire respiratory system. Once the nervous mechanism has been triggered off nothing can stop it. This reaction entails a sudden contraction of the diaphragm and the movement of certain facial muscles. In fact, a very weak local stimulus is sufficient to cause a violent reaction quite out of proportion to the stimulus. In

[*]   cf. Ida and Pingala, Section 24, pp. 144-148.

[**]   The study of conditioned reflexes by the Pavlov school, well known for its experiments with dogs, has shown that gastric juices are secreted at the same time as saliva.

the case of an allergy the cause may be even slighter – certain flower pollens, for example. But the inhalation of pure air through the nostrils is not a brusque reaction; it is a pleasant sensation of opening up to the outside world, an acceptance of our vital element, the air.

It is as if the opening of the nostrils conditions the receptivity of the whole respiratory system during inhalation. During your breathing exercises and throughout the practice of pranayama you should train yourself to inhale actively by dilating the nostrils. This advice is valid for all pranayama exercises, including alternate breathing, although in this case, obviously, only the nostril that is not closed will dilate. The perception of fresh air passing into the nostrils is thus enhanced, facilitating the necessary concentration of the mind on the process of absorbing prana.

It is, of course, impossible to breathe like this throughout the day, but with regular practice in taking the air in this way - constant training helps – the nostrils will regain their mobility. In time, the habit of our ancestors, lost through what we pompously call 'civilisation', will re-establish itself, at least partially, throughout the day and even at night.

Even if the change is imperceptible, it is not too optimistic to say that it can increase the amount of inhaled air by 10 per cent. At eighteen breaths per minute, this represents half a million litres more air per annum entering our lungs and invigorating their cells.[*] Experiment by alternating normal breathing with breathing in which you actively take the air. You will soon be convinced of the effectiveness of the latter.

You will also notice that only active 'taking the air' makes breathing easy, harmonious and well balanced, which is always desirable but particularly so during pranayama exercises.

---

[*] Even when breathing very lightly (500 cc per inhalation), about 5 million litres of air reach the lungs each year.

In this section we shall consider in detail that underestimated organ, the nose. We have already mentioned its role in prana absorption, but we shall now return to the same question, but from a different angle, that is in connection with the sense of smell. It is a very special sense.

The sensory life of the ant, and consequently the content of its psyche, consists almost exclusively of olfactory sensations. Its antennae, specialised in the perception of different smells, make it possible for the ant to follow traces. Its road is sign posted with smells. It is by smell, moreover, that it identifies its friends and locates its enemies, noses out its eggs and recognises its nest. The brain of the ant is primitive, but in many mammals, some of which are very close to ourselves, we find a very highly developed sense of smell. Think of the dog.

The importance of the role of olfactory sensations to an animal is related to the surface available for perceiving such sensations. The olfactory mucous membrane of the dog covers practically the whole of the complicated labyrinth which forms its nose. Indeed, this surface when spread out is almost half as large as the same dog's coat. In man, on the other hand, this zone is tiny, hardly the area of a postage stamp.

In civilised man the role of the sense of smell is becoming smaller and smaller. It seems that as man becomes more intellectual and more civilised, sight and hearing increase in importance to the detriment of the other senses, particularly the sense of smell. In the animal the sense of smell helps it to find its prey and to be aware of its enemies, and stimulates the sexual reflex. The odour given off by certain female butterflies attracts the male, sometimes from many miles away. This gives some idea of the enormous sensitivity of certain species to smells. Although the importance of the sense of smell has diminished in man, deep ties continue to exist and are fixed in the very structure of our brain. It is therefore indispensable to bear this in mind in the study and practice of pranayama techniques.

In the process of evolution the human brain has grown like a town which has developed progressively. There is the old city with its old districts (the palaeocortex) and the new part of the town (the neocortex) . The very sensitive nerve endings which cover the relatively small olfactory area in the nose are directly connected to the 'old city', the cerebral structures we have inherited from our most distant ancestors. By reflex we reach this 'visceral brain' and through it such organs as the heart, the blood vessels, the bladder, the intestines, the gall bladder, the pupils, etc. Through other connections we influence the pituitary gland and thus, by hormonal routes, the whole endocrine system, our chemical nervous system.

In order to breathe correctly during pranayama we need to know the 'aerodynamic' peculiarities of our nose. The air current which enters the nose is divided into three streams in each nostril (see diagram). In the olfactory region at the top of the nasal cavity the direction of the air flow is reversed, bringing the air into contact with zones able to distinguish smells. In normal respiration only an extremely small part of the air comes into contact with the olfactory zone, yet it is possible to direct a considerable stream of air consciously towards it. This is what we must do in order to grasp the greatest possible quantity of prana and increase the efficiency of pranayama exercises.

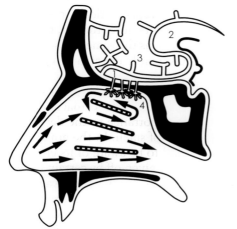

1 olfactory nerve endings (peduncles)
2 callosum
3 brain
4 olfactory fibres

The arrows show the direction of the three streams of inhaled air. Note that the direction of flow is reversed in the region covered by the olfactory fibres. Note also the direct connection between these fibres and the brain.

We already know the exercise in which we inhale while imagining that we are smelling a rose; the air flow is automatically slowed down and directed to this ultrasensitive region. This happens in all pranayama exercises where breathing is slowed down. But there is another means of intensifying the air flow and consequently the absorption of prana and the efficiency of pranayama. What does a dog do when it is following a scent? It sniffs. By inhaling in this jerky manner the dog directs a greatly increased flow of scent-laden air to the olfactory region.

Kapalabhati and Bhastrika have a similar effect. The rapid inversion and the increase in the respiratory flow create a turbulence in this strategic region, stimulating and toning up the whole 'visceral brain'. However, we must slow the air down at the glottis, directing it there consciously; this makes a characteristic noise. We now understand even better the importance of alternate breathing, which aims at stimulating equally the left nostril (Ida) and the right (Pingala).

The sense of smell opens the door to the deepest psychic levels, and it might be useful to mention here the use of certain scents to create 'states of mind'. For thousands of years women have used perfumes to make themselves attractive. In India, sandalwood sticks (dhoop) burn in every temple as an essential accompaniment to meditation and pranayama.

One of the best ways of stimulating Ida and Pingala is to sniff a stick of sandalwood, or simply to practice alternate breathing while smelling a real flower, preferably a rose or a lily of the valley. It is sufficient to concentrate on the smell for the mind to become completely absorbed in the act of breathing. Thus the intellect, normally so closely bound to visual and auditory impressions, is 'switched off. This is why it is preferable to practice pranayama with the eyes closed.

It is very easy to modify consciously the distribution of the air circulating in the nostrils and to direct a larger part of it to the olfactory region.

The position of the nostrils not only facilitates a better balance of air but also allows us to direct it to the olfactory region, our prana accumulator. Consider the rose again; we can reduce its scent at will by directing the air into the lower passages or increase it by guiding it towards the top of the nasal cavity. If we concentrate the mind on this region we become more clearly conscious of the odours; the conscious self enters into direct contact with the region and new lines of communication open in the sympathetic nervous system.

This way of breathing – directing the air towards the olfactory region – can also be practiced during relaxation exercises. Lying on the left side the student concentrates on the right nostril and directs the maximum amount of air there. He does the same with the left nostril while lying on the right side.

Part 2

PRANAYAMA:
PRINCIPLES AND PRACTICE

9 | The Length of Breath

Particular types of breathing correspond to each of our activities. We know without being a yogi that we breathe differently when running or relaxing, when awake or asleep.

Yogis who have studied the matter have found that there are subtle correlations between our breathing and our physical, intellectual and emotional activities. An angry man does not breathe in the same way as an anxious man; a happy and cheerful person's breathing differs from that of a neurotic. Yogis need only to watch how people breathe to know their physical and psychological condition.

The rishis of ancient India studied the various aspects of breathing: length, rhythm, duration, amplitude, centre of gravity, etc. First we shall deal with the 'length' of breath. How can it be measured? The traditional yogic method consists of moistening your palm and holding it up under your nostrils. As you exhale you will feel the air blowing on your palm and the evaporation of the moisture will cause a sensation of coolness. Then slowly move your hand away until you no longer feel the exhaled air. Thus, by measuring the distance between palm and nostrils, you obtain the approximate length of your breath. An even more accurate measurement can be achieved by suspending a tuft of cotton wool on a silk thread in front of your nostrils, gradually moving it away until it stops moving. In this way yogis have measured the average length in fingers (i.e. finger breadths) for the most diverse activities, from running to the state of samadhi.

In the Gheranda Samitha, one of the classical yoga treatises, Rishi Gherand says (verses 84–96):

'The body measures 96 fingers [about one metre 80 cm]. When exhaling, the stream of air roundly measures 12 fingers [about 20 cm from nose to hand]. When singing, its length increases to 16 fingers; when walking, to 24 fingers; when sleeping, to 30 fingers; during sexual intercouse, to 36 fingers. During strenuous exercises, to even more. By gradually shortening the natural length [i.e. distance] of the exhalation, we increase our vitality, whereas lengthening the exhalation reduces vitality .'

Moreover, the rishis noticed that the more engrossed and concentrated one is mentally, the 'shorter' the breath; in the state of samadhi it becomes imperceptible.

In order to obtain a maximum state of concentration, yoga recommends that we should become aware of our breath and gradually reduce its length. In practice, sit down in your favourite posture, spine straight and head well poised. Relax and sit motionless. Make yourself aware of your breathing; second by second, without distraction, follow the inhalation and the exhalation. During the full and deep inhalation, feel the air enter the nostrils and go down through the larynx, the throat and the bronchial tubes as deep as possible. When exhaling, slow down the stream of air coming out of the nostrils, shorten the length of breath. Breathing should become increasingly quiet and gentle, slower and slower while remaining deep. There should be no jerkiness. In this way gaseous and pranic exchanges take place under the best conditions.

Concentration is essential: do not let any worries distract you. You will justly object that this is difficult. Repeat a mantra. For Westerners I recommend 'pranava', the silent, mental repetition of 'OM'. To begin with, repeat it aloud five times, making the 'O' vibrate in both chest and throat during half the exhalation and the 'M' in the cranium (see *Yoga Self-Taught* Chapter 7. Decrease the sound until it becomes inaudible, then repeat mentally. This mental 'OM' has more psychic and pranic effect than the spoken 'OM'.

Continue in this way, gradually reducing the length of the breath. With total concentration let your mind become deeply absorbed in the 'OM'; let your mind, your breath and the 'OM' mingle with one another until they become one. Do not pause for any length of time between inhalation and exhalation. If you prolong this exercise, you may become drowsy and doze off. This is an unimportant technical hitch which can and should be avoided. One of the purposes of this exercise is to produce a controlled levelling of the subconscious. Actually one should attain a state of apparent sleep without any break in consciousness.

At this point colours or swirling lights may sometimes appear. Do not let it surprise or worry you: these luminous impressions result from the activity of the subconscious. Do not seek or reject them but remain neutral towards them. These phenomena are quite rare but must be mentioned here so that you are not disturbed if they occur.

With lungs empty, calmly hold your breath and concentrate on the sacrum at the base of the spine. While holding your breath, you can easily focus your consciousness on that spot. You may notice some vibrations.

Now imagine that you are sending a current of prana, materialising in the form of light and heat, to this area. After some practice you will definitely have a sensation of heat there, possibly also a tingling sensation. If nothing special is felt, this does not mean that the exercise is ineffective. Continue practising and the effects will not fail to occur eventually.

During inhalation make your consciousness rise along your spine; imagine that the heat is moving upwards with it. The effect is that prana, which obeys the mind as we have seen before, moves along your spine. Do not allow the exercise to be interrupted abruptly; if possible, practise somewhere where there is no risk of being disturbed. To return to a normal waking state, go through the cycle in reverse: begin with the inward pronunciation of the 'OM', then say it aloud five times, and then gradually change your breath to its normal length.

This practice is very effective and harmless; there is no risk involved in holding your breath with lungs empty. Its psychic effects are deep. The absorption of mental consciousness dims the intellect and at the same time develops intuition.

A regular five-minute practice every day, preferably at sunrise and sunset, will calm your mind and a new serenity will brighten your day. You will also notice important pranic effects. Released at the base of the spine and guided along it, prana brings permanent life and dynamism without any adverse effects to the most vital nerve centres.

10 | Jala Neti, the Nasal Douche

Neti, the method of cleansing the nose by drawing up water from an ordinary bowl, is certainly the closest to original yoga techniques. Living near to watercourses and springs the yogis and rishis of ancient India had probably begun by sniffing water up into their nostrils from their cupped hands. Later they used a bowl and adopted the technique described in *Yoga Self-Taught* Chapter 5 . Finally, as yoga was perfected, its techniques became more elaborate and yogis developed a suitable container called a 'lota', which looks like a teapot, in order to perform Jala Neti. This method is very easy and pleasant.

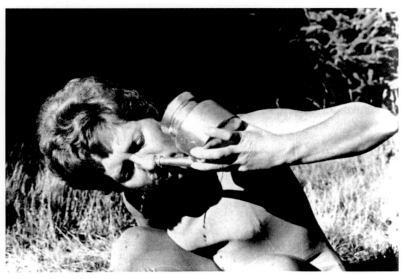

The inclination of the head is important for the successful performance of Jala Neti

Technique
Fill the lota with salted water. Some yogis use water as warm as can be tolerated; others use water at room temperature or even cold water. Each method has its advantages. Very warm water loosens the mucus better and faster, while cold water is invigorating and toughening. It

is a matter of individual preference. For a normal lota (holding a half-litre) use one level teaspoon of salt. To perform Jala Neti put the spout of the lota into the left nostril. Tilt your head to the right and let the water flow into the nostril; it will flow out of the other nostril. The conical spout will close the nostril into which it has been inserted. *Important*: during the whole operation the mouth must remain open and relaxed, whether breathing or not.

When half the water has been used, put the spout into the other nostril and repeat. If you have no lota you can perform Jala Neti with a teapot; but if the spout is too wide do not try to insert it, place it against the opening of the nostril only.

Drying the nostrils. It is necessary to dry the nostrils and the back of the throat after Jala Neti. Tilt your head forward and allow the remaining water to run out. The drying is then done by ventilation. Bend forward from the waist and hold your right wrist behind your back with your left hand. With the head bent forward, exhale forcefully through both nostrils. Raise your head and inhale, immediately expelling the air with force through both nostrils. Repeat this with your head bent to the right and then to the left (this may be reversed). For one or two minutes follow this sequence: head down, head up, bent to one side and then to the other, until the nostrils are completely dry. This method may be used for any type of Neti.

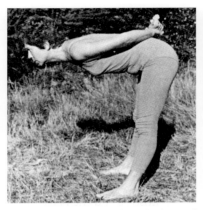

Drying the nostrils is very important; expel the air with force while raising your head.

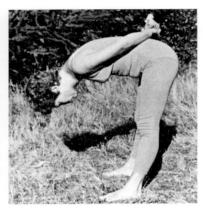

Lower your head

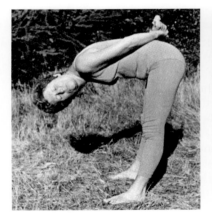

Then turn it to the left

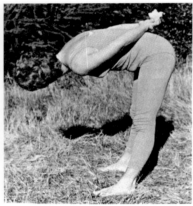

and finally to the right. Repeat these movements for at least one minute

11 | Do We Have a Pranic Body?

In esoteric yoga literature terms like 'astral body' or 'ethereal body' and similar obscure expressions are often used; they puzzle the uninitiated because they are seldom precisely defined. I shall nevertheless venture to give a definition, but first I want to eliminate such terms as 'astral body', which is quite vague and evokes the image of a ghost performing evolutions among the stars. The idea of a 'double' is not much better; it will seem incongruous to the rational reader, and 'ethereal' has no meaning for him either. I prefer the expression 'pranic body' for 'body' implies something material and 'pranic' also takes us back to the plane of physical phenomena. It is by no means perfect but, for lack of a better term, I shall use it.

Before going any further, let us sum up what we have established so far. Prana with a capital 'P' comprises the sum total of all forces manifest in the universe, and prana with a small 'p' signifies their specialised and limited manifestations. We have detected certain forms of prana, that of air in particular. We know that prana manifests itself in our bodies in a variety of ways: our nervous energy, which is of an electric nature, is a good example. We know that energy currents run through our bodies without following the nerve channels.* These currents probably correspond to the meridians of acupuncture, a therapy whose efficacy is no longer questioned. The 'pranic body' is the sum of the subtle forces produced, assimilated and carried in our physical systems. Let us examine the details.

We shall imitate those Indian thinkers who use analogies in order to define abstract concepts. These analogies often give us sufficiently precise insight into phenomena which otherwise would be difficult to understand.

So let us compare the human being to a submarine; the skin represents the armour plating, the organs represent the machinery, and the brain is the command post. The nerves represent the electric cables that pass through the vessel. The ship is matter; the strength of its steel shows us that it is real. Likewise, our dense physical body (bones, flesh, etc.) is composed of material, solid particles. But the submarine

---

* This subject will be considered more fully in Section 23

also has a 'pranic' body.

Reduced to its solid components, the machine is just an inert, motionless mass. It only becomes operational when certain forces run through it, when an electric current travels from the generator to the engines which make the propellors turn, or along the internal telephone lines which link the various posts and parts of the ship and transmit orders or steer the rudder. The sum of these forces, which are mainly of a purely electric nature, 'doubles' the vessel and forms its 'pranic' body which is almost intangible. The 'pranic double' of the submarine is not the same as the 'tangible body', just as the electric current cannot be identified with its conducting wires. Yet there is a bond between them, an interaction. The wires have an effect on the current since they carry it, but, whereas the dense physical body of the ship can be touched, seen and weighed, its pranic body is not directly perceived by the senses: it becomes visible only through its manifestations (motion, for example) or is revealed by devices such as voltmeters. This subtle or pranic body actually manipulates the dense body from which it partly originates, since the generators (which are material) produce the current from fuel oil which is also both tangible and visible.

So it is within our body. Food is transformed into prana, or rather it constitutes one of the sources of prana. All these forces running through our body form our subtle or pranic 'body' which actually manipulates our dense body, which is sometimes called 'gross'. Although there is no identity between the gross and the pranic bodies, there is both interpenetration and interaction.

The ship gets in touch with the surrounding universe through its pranic body. Through the radar of our sense organs pictures from the outside world appear on the screen of our consciousness: obstacles, enemy ships, allied aeroplanes, which the officer on watch (the vigilant inner self) studies; from all these data he determines the actions and reactions of the ship. The radio receivers and transmitters put it in touch with other ships and with general headquarters.

At the command of the inner self and in agreement with it, the conscious self regulates all the moves of the warship, decides whether it must remain in port or get under way and, if the latter, in which direction. Likewise, our pranic and physical bodies penetrate each other. The former is the real animator but remains, in a subtle way, an instrument in the service of the 'self.

Now we come to the question: are there illnesses of pranic origin? If the submarine has a pranic body is it not possible for this body to show some kind of disturbance? A lowering of the electric potential may reduce the power of the engines considerably and it could upset the radar or the radio system. The causes may be physical – such as a short-circuit of the wires, or unsuitable fuel which interferes with the normal functioning of the generator and with the production of the necessary current (prana). Similarly, insufficient or unsuitable nourishment (in its broadest meaning, since air is one of its main components) may effect our pranic body and upset the functioning of the physical body, though some disturbances may be of a purely pranic nature. In this case, remedies meant to cure physical ailments will have no effect except perhaps to change the location of the problem. How many illnesses that have been 'cured' by a specific chemical drug reappear elsewhere in a different form! 'It's nerves,' we say. Should we not consider the possibility of disturbances of a pranic nature and apply pranic remedies? Is it not by their effect on the pranic body that acupuncture needles disperse or invigorate the excess of yang or yin and so cure some illnesses that have resisted other treatment? To return to our analogy: pranic disturbances may also be caused by wrong manoeuvres on the part of the navigating officer. Mental trouble, too, may affect physical health; this has been confirmed by psychosomatic medicine. In any case, pranayama does not have a therapeutic goal; its sole goal is to guarantee the integrity and equilibrium of the pranic body, to make sure that it constantly receives the necessary supply of prana, and to control it and accumulate it. All in all, its role is to transform the 'dense body – subtle body' complex into an instrument of self-fulfilment. This is the purpose of the exercises already described. They are far more than a simple method of breathing, whose only purpose is to ensure a sufficient supply of oxygen. Beyond this energy balance the self also has at its disposal all the controls of the remarkably complex machinery of a living body – from the simplest to the most complex, from amoeba to man. Through our pranic or spiritual body we must control the physical body and make it act in accordance not only with the orders of the deep ego but also with those of the self. This power is obtained consciously and with increased efficiency by yogis using the methods of pranayama and concentration. The observation of pranic effect of practising asanas shows the profound unity of yoga. Exercises to control the breath are not the only ones to act on the pranic body, which is also affected by asanas. If a yogi wishes to stress the difference between gymnastics and sport on the one hand and yoga on the other, he says: 'Gymnastics cause an expenditure of prana, while yoga asanas regulate the flow of prana and accumulate it in the body.'

Indeed, one *should* feel rested and full of energy after a session of asanas performed correctly, unless there is a fault in the technique. Postures affect the pranic body directly, which explains their remarkable efficiency. Yet externally nothing spectacular seems to happen since the body is either motionless or moves only slowly. This is why pranayama exercises acquire their full meaning and efficiency only when combined with the yoga postures.

12 | Nadi Sodhana, the Purifying Breath

In the preceding section I defined the concept of the pranic body which is composed of the entirety of the spiritual forces (nervous and otherwise) active in our bodies. This energy body guarantees the cohesion of the more compact particles of our material, visible body. It represents our vital force. Let us pursue our analogy with the warship: we know that electric power runs through the ship along tangible conductors, the electric cables and telephone wires. Electric power can sometimes do without conductors, as in the walkie-talkie, radar or the ship's radio. Similarly, energy does not wander haphazardly in our body; it follows well-defined paths and it is channelled and guided. But just as conductors (electric cables or telephone wires) must not be confused with electricity itself, the energy circulating in our bodies must not be confused with their conductors, the *nadis*.

Nadis

What are these conductors, the nadis? According to yoga anatomy, our bodies contain a complex network of 72,000 nadis – literally 'tubes' in Sanskrit – through which our energy flows. Some authors identify the nadis with our nerves, whereas others consider them spiritual and imperceptible to our senses, though nonetheless material. The supporters of the 'nadis-nerves' theory state that in old, classical treatises rishis describe the nadis as tubes consisting of three layers. The inner layer is called *sira*, the middle one *damani* and the outer one *nadi*, the same word as is used to describe the whole organ. We must admit that electric wires and nerves have a similar structure, consisting of superimposed sheaths. For more details see Section 24, p. 144.

Yogis state that in the average man a number of these conductors cannot be permeated by pranic forces and consequently energy can only circulate through the body badly. Since prana is the principal motive force of our whole physical and mental life, this condition creates various psycho-physiological disorders. One of the prime objectives of yoga is to ensure a free circulation of pranic forces at all levels. This is why the rishis emphasised the need for an appropriate diet, for asanas which keep a maximum number of nadis open, and for a healthy and simple life, if possible mostly in the open air. The practice of yoga described in *Yoga Self-Taught* and in *Je perfectionne mon yoga* enables a Westerner to maintain the permeability of a sufficient number of nadis and guarantees a correct energy metabolism sufficient to meet ordinary needs. However, pranayama is indispensable to attain this dynamic state of both mental and physical health. The first prerequisite is to make sure that the nadi distribution network is capable of playing its part.

Ida and Pingala
Among the spiritual conductors, yogis distinguish two main ones which will be described later at length and which are called Ida and Pingala. Here we only need to know that Ida represents the energy conductor starting at the left nostril and Pingala its right counterpart. These nadis or conductors travel the length of the spine and, according to some yoga traditions, cross each other several times running through the main *chakras* . Each nostril plays a unique role; they are not interchangeable. It is essential that both are free and clear. This is the reason why the nasal douche or Neti should be performed before beginning pranayama exercises.

In spite of this cleansing, one or other nostril is often blocked; this is quite normal. Yogis, who are keen observers, have noted that this happens with alternate nostrils, and that the obstruction passes from one nostril to the other approximately every two hours. Modern medicine is well aware of this phenomenon. It is called 'alternate rhinitis', as one nostril becomes free when the other becomes obstructed. This alternation occurs continuously during the day with lesser or greater intensity, depending on the vital equilibrium and particularly on the condition of the liver. Alternate rhinitis is therefore a normal phenomenon which usually goes unnoticed. Even if there is no stoppage, one nostril is usually freer than the other. To test this, use the technique mentioned on p.55, Section 9; moisten your palm and put it near one nostril and then near the other. You are bound to notice the difference. If you want to see the difference between the two air currents, bring your nose near to a mirror. Exhale normally and watch the two uneven rings which have formed on it.

How can one clear the nostrils? Except in cases of physical obstruction such as mucus (which should be removed by Neti), polyps or an abnormally positioned septum, there are many yoga techniques for clearing the nostrils (I know at least eight of them), but in practice it is enough if you know two or three. The first one is a little slower than the others but it is simple, easy and foolproof. If your left nostril is stopped up, lie down on your right side and relax. After between one and three minutes you will notice that the stopped-up nostril is clearing itself up and the air is passing freely, while the other remains clear. Concentrating on the stopped-up nostril will speed up the process. Note that Ida is the left, cooling nostril, while Pingala is the right, warming one. According to yoga tradition, one should breathe through the right nostril at night, which means sleeping on your left side. Many people are reluctant to do this out of fear of pressure on the heart. This fear is unfounded; the heart is situated almost in the middle of the chest. Swami Sivananda used to say that food was easier to digest this way and, as a doctor, he did not make this statement lightly but based it on physiological facts. Actually the stomach is better supported and functions more normally when we lie on the left side.

The second technique is as follows: find a spot at the back of the neck near the base of the skull and press it with your thumb. It is easy to find, and a gentle but firm pressure on this spot will clear up the nostril, even if you are getting a cold in the head – to which you should, as a practising yogi, be immune anyway. This method works even faster than the first provided you find the exact spot.

The third method is the fastest of all. In India, the equipment of a perfect yogi includes a short crutch. All you do is place the fork under the opposite armpit and lean on it for a few seconds. In Western countries, where this tool is not available, press the armpit firmly on the back of a chair. The right spot is easily found as it is particularly tender.

The most efficient classical exercise for purifying the nadis is called Nadi Shodana Pranayama. This alternate breathing – *without* holding the breath – is used to balance and equalise the pranic current flowing through the nose and to purify the whole network of the nadis. Otherwise, pranayama loses much of its efficiency. At the beginning of the exercise the air current need not be identical on both sides. Only a severe blocking of the nose can prevent you from practising it. In that case first clear the nostril with the help of one of the techniques above.

Before detailing the exercise we must know how to regulate the alternation of breathing; then we must learn how to clear the nostrils and how to close them correctly in order to practise alternate breathing. First we must know how to place the fingers. Open your right hand and bend the index and middle fingers against your palm. The thumb is used for closing the right nostril while the fourth and fifth fingers will take care of the left nostril. The first picture shows how (see p. 70).

Put the right thumb against the soft flesh at the end of the nostril to close it. Practise pressing the fourth and fifth finger against the left nostril. It is important that only the fingertips touch the nose, never the nails. Now begin the exercise: posture as usual, straight spine, relaxed attitude, concentrate.

1   *Exhale slowly and deeply* without closing the nostrils but be ready to do so.
2   *Inhale slowly and quietly through* the left nostril while closing the right.
3   *At the end of the inhalation* close both nostrils. Hold your breath for not more than one or two seconds.
4   Keep the left nostril closed and *exhale through the right as quietly as possible*.
5   When the lungs are empty inhale slowly and quietly *through the right nostril*.
6   Close both nostrils and wait for a second, then open the left nostril and exhale slowly and silently.
7   Inhale through the same nostril and continue.

To sum up:
1   Exhale on the left
2   Inhale on the left
3   Exhale on the right
4   Inhale on the right
5   Exhale on the left
6   Inhale on the left... etc.

Concentration
At first your attention will be absorbed by the movement of your fingers and by the alternation of closing and opening the nostrils. What seems complicated at the beginning soon becomes simple and logical. When you no longer need to think about your fingers, concentrate upon the air passing through your nostrils; if you can, visualise prana as already indicated.

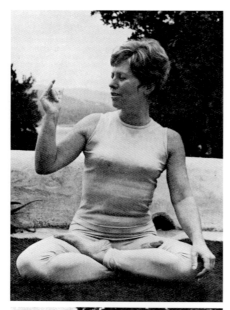

Bend the second and third fingers. The thumb will close the right nostril; the fourth and fifth fingers will close the left nostril.

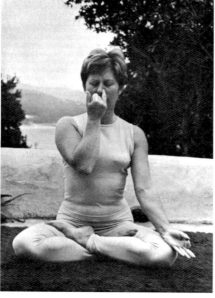

Alternate breathing is a basic pranayama exercise. Do it every day.

The best time and how long for

Morning and evening are equally suitable. There is one absolute rule: never practise immediately after a meal, but wait for at least half an hour.

You may prolong the exercise as much as you wish provided you do not feel tired. Weariness will not affect your lungs, but it will affect your arm and your mind. To prevent your arm from getting tired, hold it against your body. You will soon find the best and least tiring position. If, after two or three minutes, your face feels hot, it indicates that cell breathing has been stimulated and that one of the goals of the exercise has been attained: recharging your cellular batteries with fresh prana. The regular practice of this exercise purifies your nadis in a few weeks. With the first serious and regular attempts you can feel the benefit of the exercise, which is not dangerous if performed in an easy, unhurried way and in a quiet place.

Ratio between exhalation and inhalation

At first do not try to establish a ratio; just make sure you slow down your breathing. When the exercise has become familiar, *even up* the length of exhalation and inhalation. Persevere until the equilibrium between them becomes automatic and easy; only then go on to more advanced exercises.

Summary

In short, we are dealing with an exercise without breath retention. Its aim is to regulate breathing in order, (a) to purify the nadis and make sure the other pranayama exercises are efficient, (b) to succeed in getting an identical flow of air (and therefore of prana) on each side by alternately closing the nostrils, and (c) to equalise the lengths of exhalation and inhalation.

Avoid any muscular contraction of the face, particularly round the eyes, on the forehead, the lips and the chin; do not clench your teeth; relax your jaws, tongue, throat and neck. The lips, though relaxed, remain closed. Close your eyes during the exercise.

'Tsamin sari svasa prasvasa yorgati viccedha pranayama.' (Pranayama is the interruption of inhalation and exhalation when it [the asana] has been mastered.) Patanjali, 'Aphorisms on Yoga'; see *Les Yogas pratiques* by Vivekananda.

This quotation indicates the fundamental importance of breath retention in pranayama. In fact breath retention is its very essence and other techniques serve only to prepare for it and support it.

If there is any section in this book that should be studied thoroughly this is it; by explaining the consequences of breath retention it shows that it can be incorporated in one's personal practice without harm. Quite the contrary: physical health and psychic dynamism will benefit immensely.

Yogis are able to hold their breath for several minutes (up to half an hour or more) without any harmful effects, a fact which puzzles our physiologists. But yogis do not perform these feats merely to astonish physiologists but rather to control prana and for their action on the mind. The techniques are so far removed from the idea of a performance that their very existence has remained secret for thousands of years. For yogis, therefore, pranayama begins with (but is more than) breath retention, or at least with exercises involving holding the breath in a more or less prolonged manner. But Westerners should not get carried away: breath retention requires serious preparation and the exercises given in earlier sections form its basis. In view of its important psycho-physiological reactions, caution – but not cowardice – is indispensable. What goes on when the breath is held must be precisely understood, especially in the absence of a qualified teacher.

First let us examine the purely physiological effects by referring to the great exponents who are able to hold their breath for thirty minutes or more, the seals and walruses. These animals are of great interest to us because, despite differences of shape, way of life, etc., they are mammals whose physiology is comparable to ours.

So why is it that we cannot normally hold our breath for more than between twenty-five and seventy-five seconds, except for trained divers or sponge and pearl fishers who can continue for as long as three or four minutes, the equivalent of only 10 per cent of a walrus's ability? There is only one other mammal that can compete with the walrus: the sloth, that toothless mammal that lives in the Brazilian forests, has only two fingers on each hand, lives suspended from branches and owes its name to the slowness of its movements. This fact – the ability of a few mammals to hold their breath for long periods – intrigues the biologists, excites their curiosity and encourages research into what they call an 'immersion reflex'. The sea elephant came to their rescue and enabled them to throw some light on such phenomena. This creature, which can reach a length of eighteen feet and weigh a ton, is among the largest of living mammals and is found off the coasts of Mexico and Guadeloupe. A team of American scientists, including the famous physiologist Per Scholander of the Scripps Institute of Oceanography, his colleague Merrill Spencer and an engineer, Marcus Intaglietta, tackled the problem. In February 1964 some sea elephants were captured off Guadeloupe and experiments followed, during which a captured animal would be tied to a weighted plank while instruments were connected to a fin artery in order to check its physiological reactions. The sea elephant was then immersed in a tank of water (males as well as females were studied). By forcing it to remain under the water for ten, twenty or even thirty minutes, it was observed that the diving reflex was fully released after only a few immersions; to all appearances it took a seal a certain time to understand that the experiment was like a real immersion, said Spencer. The instruments showed that the heartbeats were slowed down drastically as soon as the 'reflex' was released (that is as soon as the nose of the seal was under water). The normal pulse-beat of a seal out of water is between eighty and ninety per minute, but it falls immediately to twelve a minute during immersion, which corresponds to a sharp reduction of the circulation in order to economise the oxygen carried by the blood. Such a decrease in circulation could harm the heart and especially the brain, where any prolonged lack of oxygen causes lesions, sometimes fatal and always irreversible. Research has shown that the capillaries in the tail and the fins of the seal almost close to concentrate the oxygen-laden blood on the organs needing it most: the heart and the brain. The seal releases the oxygen stored in its muscles, where it is usually kept in large quantities, to supply its extremities. Another major observation was that during immersion the seal modified its metabolism by the partial break-up of sugars to produce energy without depleting its limited oxygen reserves. This 'immersion reflex' is being studied by Western scientists for possible application to humans. Nowadays it is not only the oxygen supply of sponge and pearl fishers which may be cut during their professional work. Men in submarines, pilots of supersonic airplanes, and cosmonauts all risk having their oxygen supply cut off entirely from one moment to the next. If man, too, were able to employ the immersion reflex he could gain precious minutes, which might mean the difference between life and death. Science has found that man has in fact a rudimentary immersion reflex, atrophied perhaps by lack of use but which could be developed. Scientists asked an old pearl diver to immerse his head in a bucket of water; his pulse rate, too, reduced to twelve beats a minute, at which point the experimenter pulled the man's head out to inquire if he felt well. If, on the other hand, the diver had blocked his nostrils in order to hold his breath without water immersion, the reduction in his pulse rate would have been less. The researchers therefore came to the conclusion that psychological facts played an important role in the release of this reflex, as even with the sea elephant it only functioned when the animal realised that it had to behave in a certain way when it was forced to accept a long immersion.

To return to pranayama: our first conclusion is that the long breath retention of yogis can be explained physiologically. Remember that holding the breath sets in action a psycho-physiological reflex which exists in a rudimentary state in humans and which can be developed. Now we face the question: why and how?

The aims of Kumbhaka

The answer cannot be simple, for the techniques of pranayama relate to the whole area of psycho-physiology. To simplify and rationalise our study let us consider the immediate objectives so as to pass on thereafter to the effects and the loftier aims. With the Hatha yogi breath retention first of all effects a decrease in the energy, the prana in his body, which is followed by a better distribution of prana throughout the whole body. The yogi seeks to acquire the power of directing more prana at will to those parts of his body where he feels it is needed.

Stimulation of the intracellular breathing

The immediate object of the various pranayama exercises with breath retention is to stimulate the inner breathing. It is good to remember that there are two kinds of breathing:

1 *Breathing through the lungs or external breathing.* This includes the nervous and muscular mechanisms which are needed to allow the outer air to penetrate to the lungs, the exchange processes in the alveoli and the expulsion of used air. The outer respiration has only two phases: inhalation and exhalation. The yogis introduced two more phases and breathing is now composed of four phases, as follows:

a   Rechaka – exhalation (the most important phase)
b   Kumbhaka with empty lungs
c   Puraka – inhalation (the effectiveness of which depends on the first phase)
d   Kumbhaka with full lungs.

The various pranayama exercises originate from modifications in each of these phases. From a pranayama viewpoint retention phases are physiologically and psychologically the most important, the rest having meaning only in relation to them.

2 *Internal or cellular breathing.* This is the only true breathing – though little known – since it constitutes the real goal of external breathing and takes place in every cell. Any cell which is in contact with oxygen absorbs it; through oxidation of some cellular elements energy is released and produces CO_2 (carbon dioxide), which the cell expels. The primary object of pranayama is to stimulate cellular breathing with increased production of internal heat by an activation of intracellular combustion. Exercises should therefore be carried out until profuse perspiration occurs. In fact, we do not perspire as fast in our temperate climates as in India, and to do so we must produce a definite rise in body temperature. The result is a 'magnetisation' of the body, a revitalisation through the activation of the biological processes of intracellular breathing. The energy, the prana thus released, is available for high psycho-physiological purposes which will be mentioned later. A sedentary Westerner living in the still air of a closed dwelling seldom has the opportunity to activate cellular breathing, which suddenly stimulates and accelerates the normal and vital processes on all the cells of the body. Regular practice ensures a good physiological

dynamism, improving the vital tonus and enabling us to withstand all the stresses and trials of life. It is not a fillip or an artificial stimulation but a deep revitalisation.

The gradations

The effects as well as the dangers of retention depend on the duration of breath-holding. We shall therefore examine the various degrees of Kumbhaka with full lungs and then discuss its effects.

1   *Kumbhaka of between three and twenty seconds.* The main effect of this type of retention, which is within everybody's reach, is to permit a better utilisation and 'digestion' of the inhaled air. If we collect and analyse exhaled air (normal breathing) we find that only 6 per cent of the 21 per cent of oxygen contained in the inhaled air is actually absorbed into the system. In fact, it is because exhaled air still contains between 14 and 15 per cent oxygen that a victim can be revived by mouth-to-mouth resuscitation. By lengthening the air contact with the pulmonary membrane, exchanges are effected in the best conditions: the oxygen absorption is increased while, at the same time, carbon dioxide (CO_2) evacuation is more complete.

In this way breathing is performed with maximum benefit. This type of Kumbhaka may be practised at any time: it has no counter-indications and constitutes the indispensable preparation for the next step.

2   *Kumbhaka of between twenty and ninety seconds.* When breath retention lasts more than twenty seconds, it creates much more pronounced reactions. It is not dangerous if it is performed according to the instructions described in detail in the section on exercises. A Westerner should in principle not go beyond this stage – with few exceptions, when guided by a qualified instructor. Breath retention is practised until such time as reflex mechanisms dominate willpower and cause exhalation to start. Breath is held to a bearable point without any exaggerated effort of will or any violent reactions from the organism. If the progression is slow, regular and helped by daily practice, these exercises are accessible to the Westerner provided he takes some precautions and uses common sense. There are counterindications (see below).

3   *Kumbhaka of ninety seconds and up to several minutes.* In this category, the yogi reaches a controlled pre-comatose state which is accompanied by very deep physiological reactions capable of causing a complete revitalisation (probably by stimulating the formation in the system of the biostimulins discovered by Filatov). In 1933 Professor Filatov, a member of the USSR Academy of Medicine and a specialist in the grafting of the cornea, was working on a process for preserving corneas by refrigeration. He was surprised to see that the grafts which had been frozen for a long time *'revived' better than did fresh corneas.* This unexpected fact was the starting-point of systematic investigations of the phenomena which take place in living tissues during freezing on the one hand, and of the reactions of the body receiving the graft on the other. Here again research workers were surprised: the grafts had a stimulating, rejuvenating effect on the *whole* body receiving them. Filatov supposed that the graft cells subjected to the action of the cold, threatened with death, produced a stimulating substance in their struggle for survival. After long research, he formulated his famous theory: 'When tissue separated from the body is kept in unfavourable but not fatal conditions for survival its biochemical activity is modified, producing non-specific biostimulins, capable of stimulating *all* the vital reactions of the organism on which it is grafted.'

If an entire organism is placed in such 'unfavourable but not fatal' conditions will there not be a formation of biostimulins without having to separate the tissue from the organism? This hypothesis is plausible. There is no doubt that an interruption of the oxygen supply will soon create unfavourable conditions leading to asphyxia and eventually to death if prolonged. Filatov's theory would explain and make plausible the rishis' assertions that extended pranayama would be like a 'fountain of youth'. As may be surmised, such prolonged pranayama corresponds to physiological acrobatics not without danger and only to be performed under the guidance of qualified experts. When Indian yogis declare that pranayama is dangerous and must be performed with a guru present, they are referring to the advanced stages of these exercises. There are no such restrictions when retentions do not last more than two minutes. We shall therefore concentrate on Kumbhaka No. 2, the most useful for Western people.

Physiological effects of Kumbhaka No. 2
Kumbhaka No. 2 should release the immersion reflex already described

and produce some important modifications to circulation in the extremities, which is why the exercise must be performed either in the lotus, siddhasana or, at least, the diamond posture, in order to slow down the circulation in the legs to the benefit of the heart and brain. Important changes in metabolism which take place include a partial breakdown of sugar with direct formation of oxygen to compensate for the interruption of supply from outside. During breath retention the CO_2 level in the blood rises and the internal temperature tends to go up. The ventilation of the lungs plays the part of a radiator disposing of the heat produced by intracellular combustion. Just as the engine of your car would overheat without the action of the radiator, combustion in those living engines, the cells, produces heat which would overheat the system if the skin and particularly the lungs did not act as radiators. When the breath is held the pulmonary radiator is disconnected. The organism responds by asking for greater activity on the part of the skin, which explains that real feeling of warmth and perhaps perspiration. We now understand how the yogis succeed in fighting the cold by breath control, and how in 1966 Swami Dhirendra Brahmachari, Pandit Nehru's own guru, who had been invited by the Soviet Union to train cosmonauts in yoga techniques, could leave an Air India plane in Moscow in midwinter, clad in sheer muslin. The Russians who were waiting at the airport in fur-lined coats and hats and wearing gloves were astounded when they saw him on the tarmac in this outfit, smiling in the typical Moscow winter. A charitable Russian offered his coat to Dhirendra Brahmachari who refused it and said with a smile: 'I manufacture my own heat when I need it.'

Controlling the 'vital centre'

The main effects of Kumbhaka No. 2, however, are felt in the sympathetic nervous system, particularly in the respiratory centre situated in the spinal marrow, in the swelling at the base of the brain called the medula oblongata, where the 'vital centre' is found. An ordinary needle prick on that spot would be fatal. The task of the respiratory centre is to adapt the breathing to external as well as internal conditions. It is the precise and continuous resonator of the whole psycho-physiological situation. It centralises a mass of information coming from the entire body; it reacts to the slightest variations in the pH of the blood, in CO_2 level, in oxygen content, as well as in pressure in the surrounding blood vessels. The respiratory centre is part of the elongated marrow of the spine which gives it a privileged and unique position as it is linked *directly* to the whole of the nervous system. It is closely connected not only to all the centres of the marrow of the spine which commands the respiratory mechanisms but also to the pneumogastric nerve (see below), as well as the higher cerebral levels. Therefore, any modification of the outside world perceived by the senses and any change in the psychological behaviour (conscious cortical activity, intellectual work, emotions) instantaneously find an echo in the respiratory centre in order to adapt the respiratory behaviour to a given situation. In particular, every emotion modifies our respiratory rhythm and causes variations in the CO_2 of the blood content. The respiratory centre also acts on the whole blood circulation and vice versa. The slightest muscular movement alters the blood composition and effects the respiratory centre.

A peculiarity of the respiratory centre is that it usually functions autonomously, like the other sympathetic centres, but it also has the unique privilege of being able to take orders from the conscious self; it can co-operate with it. In Kumbhaka No. 2, the conscious self inhibits the reflex mechanism of the respiratory centre and imposes its will. Here is a 'technical' comparison: in everyday life the respiratory centre behaves like the automatic pilot of a commercial plane which commands all the reactions of the engine. The human pilot just has to watch the general course, but he may, if he wishes, disconnect the automatic pilot and take the controls himself. As soon as the 'conscious self' interferes with the respiratory mechanisms to slow them down, to accelerate them or to stop them, it takes on a key position.

Key to organic control
Breathing is the great borderline function which, from a physiological viewpoint, separates these two distinct areas: unconscious and reflex organic activity on one side and willed activity on the other. It is impossible to give direct orders to the liver, the stomach or the spleen, but it is possible to regulate breathing at any moment.

What happens when breathing instead of being involuntary becomes conscious? At that moment the conscious self is in direct contact with it. During Kumbhaka the conscious self enters into direct relation with the respiratory centre and takes control of the whole organism in an even more definite manner than during the conscious slowing down of breathing. After a few seconds of Kumbhaka a conflict will arise between the respiratory centre and the will of the conscious self which stops the breathing movements. After a few seconds of retention, the respiratory centre already registers changes in the composition of the blood: the CO_2 level goes up while the oxygen content goes down. The respiratory centre is excited and tries to restart the breathing movements but the conscious self opposes it. The longer it holds out the more power it will have on the respiratory centre as it masters the inhalation reflex. Stimulation of the respiratory centre will then act on the pneumogastric nerve.

Stimulation of the pneumogastric nerve
As you may recall, the autonomous nervous system is composed on the one hand of the sympathetic nerves which run along the spine with a string of ganglions close to the vertebrae. This is the action system: its activities tend to mobilise and utilise the reserves of the body for action in the outside world. On the other hand, there is the pneumogastric nerve which starts from the medulla oblongata near the respiratory centre and is the nerve centre for the pharynx, the larynx, the trachea, the lungs, the aorta, the heart, the oesophagus, the stomach, the small intestine, the pancreas, the liver, the spleen, the kidneys, the colon and the blood vessels of the viscera – in short all the organs – exactly like its antagonist, the sympathetic nervous system. The two systems are antagonistic: one plays the part of an accelerator, the other of a brake, although in some cases their roles may be reversed. The pneumogastric nerve controls organic preservation.

It is interesting to note that the average civilised man is primarily sympathicotonic, in other words his vegetative nervous system is characterised by a continuous excitement of the sympathetic nerves. This perpetual disruption of equilibrium is the cause of many symptoms that you will be able to recognise as they appear. A sympathicotonic person has dilated pupils and dry rather than shiny eyes. His mouth is dry, he is covered with cold sweat, and he may suddenly turn pale. It is the sympathetic system which makes your hair stand on end, gives you palpitations, makes your heart beat too fast. The excitation of the sympathetic nerves slows down the peristaltic movements of the digestive tract, reduces the secretion of the digestive glands, often causes spasmodic constipation and a slow and difficult digestion. Besides, he continually feels 'overexcited' because of an overproduction of adrenalin. This is the classic syndrome - which manifests itself in various degrees - of the reactions of a city dweller caught in the whirl of numerous occupations, overburdened with responsibilities or, in other words, with worries. He sleeps poorly, is on edge, feels simultaneously anxious and aggressive.

Kumbhaka will stimulate its antagonist, the pneumogastric nerve, the one which 'makes your mouth water', leaves the skin dry while allowing its normal irrigation, calms the heart, slows down the pulse, amplifies the peristaltic movements of the intestine, cures constipation and at the same time encourages the secretions of the digestive glands. While protracted breath retention stimulates the pneumogastric nerve, it restores the neuro-vegetative equilibrium. That is why the sympathicotonic individual in particular is recommended to breathe slowly, deeply and thoroughly as often as possible in order to see all the symptoms of overexcitement of the sympathetic nerve progressively disappear. Kumbhaka No. 2 constitutes for him a first-rate stabiliser.

1 4 | H o w   T o   H o l d   Y o u r   B r e a t h

Breath retention stimulates cellular breathing; it increases the pro-duction of bio-energy and pranic exchanges in the whole body and exerts a powerful effect on the neuro-vegetative system. These benefits may be secured without danger provided the following rules are observed.

1   Regular practice of the classical asanas (for example, those de-scribed in *Yoga Self-Taught*) to keep the whole spine flexible. This is why the ancient treatises (particularly the Asthanga Yoga of Patanjali) refer to the asanas as the stage preceding pranayama. Asanas quicken the circulation of the blood throughout the body, open up capillaries and enable prana, released during breath retention, to be distributed through the whole organism and to be 'dynamised without short-cir-cuits'. Prolonged breath retention may cause pranic disturbances in a body which has not been limbered up by asanas, usually characterised by a rigid spine. These disturbances have no serious consequences since everything goes back to normal the moment the pranayama exercises are stopped. It is advisable to practice pranayama (including breath retentions of more than forty seconds) after the asana session.

2   During pranayama with Kumbhaka the spine must be as straight and as vertical as possible, but the pelvic area should be tilted slightly forwards. It should not be performed lying down.

3   During breath retention Mula Bandha must take place (see page 190), in other words the anus must be contracted and raised, affecting the whole perineum. We must visualise the spine as a pile of coins, each with a hole in the centre,* through which hangs a thread. The vertebrae are the coins; the thread is the marrow. Since important pranic currents will run through the marrow, whether you are con-sci-ous of it or not, it must 'hang' freely in the spinal column.

4   Breath retention must be performed on an empty stomach. While exercises, including voluntary and slow breathing without retention, may be performed at any time of the day, pranayama with Kumbhaka may not. The time which must elapse between the last meal and the pranayama session depends, of course, on the size and composition of

---

*   After the comparison cited by Evans-Wentz in the work entitled *Bardo, the Ti-betan Book of the Dead.*

the meal and on individual peculiarities. Some people digest quickly, others, especially sympathicotonic people who derive the greatest benefit from these exercises, have slow digestions. If pranayama is practised after asanas there is no problem, as these must also be practised on an empty stomach. As an indication, this time lapse may vary from one and a half to five hours! In any case, no serious consequences are to be expected other than a temporary digestive uneasiness.

5   Progressive training is particularly important, because it is comparatively easy to hold your breath and this may encourage some untrained people to practise retention at random, leading possibly to a state of euphoria which could persist even after the exercises are ended, and this in turn could lead to an increase in the length and frequency of retention, sometimes causing fever, which could frighten the victim. I personally know of a young man who was forbidden to practise asanas because he was a hunchback, but being a yoga lover he practised concentration and meditation for one hour a day. Then he discovered in a book some pranayama exercises with breath retention which he immediately put into practice at a great rate from the first day. He experienced an extraordinary feeling of euphoria, but the next day had a temperature of 39°C. He sought my advice as he suspected that the fever had been caused by pranayama, but I was able to reassure him that stopping the exercises would bring the fever down. And it did. The condition of his spine did not allow the correct distribution of prana and this was the cause of his trouble.

A sensation of warmth is normal but it must not last for hours; it should disappear fairly soon after the end of the session. A period of heat such as this need leave no serious consequences, but it acts as a warning. The victims of these spectacular but quite harmless disturbances are often too frightened to try breath retention again, and this can all be avoided if the length and frequency of retention are increased very gradually.

6   The most common error by beginners is to 'fill up', thinking they will be able to hold out longer if they get as much air as possible into their lungs. But it is not the last inhalation which has a decisive effect on the length of retention, since the volume of oxygen held in the lungs is very small compared with that carried by the blood, whose saturation depends upon the previous breaths. Therefore, breath retention must be preceded by deep, slow and complete breathing except when practising hyperventilation exercises such as Kapalabhati and

Bhastrika (see pp 149 and 160). Pulmonary ventilation exercises cause a massive expulsion of CO_2 and must therefore be followed by breath retention in order to bring the CO_2 rate in the blood back to its normal level. It is wrong to believe that CO_2 is harmful per se; its presence is indispensable for the chemical equilibrium of the blood.

To hold the breath correctly one must take at least five complete and deep yoga breaths; during the last, which should be no longer than the rest, inhalation will gradually slow down until it becomes retention. During retention, even more than during deep breathing exercises, you should concentrate on what goes on in your body, especially in the thorax, and you must listen to your heart beats.

7   During retention all is well if, after a few seconds, your heartbeats slow down to a calm but strong rhythm. Then you become aware of the blood circulation in the form of a pulsation which seems to shake the whole thorax rhythmically. If this occurs, everything is perfect: these reactions are normal. After a period which varies greatly from one person to another, your body demands air. A beginner must not fight this urge too long and he must let exhalation begin almost imperceptibly. Some yogis recommend that a few cubic centimetres of fresh air should be inhaled immediately before starting exhalation so as to make its control easier.

8   Exhalation must be slow, continuous and thorough. When it is finished the last traces of air should be forced out by contracting the muscles of the rib-cage and the abdomen. At the end of this forced exhalation, hold your breath for two or three seconds; then let inhalation start gently. Avoid holding your breath sharply or releasing it suddenly. The transition must be smooth so that the air in your lungs is expelled gradually. If you are unable to control the exhalation or if you hold your breath until you feel you are about to burst, you have exceeded your capabilities. All the phases must be controlled, including exhalation and the subsequent inhalation. If you are forced to inhale too fast after a hasty exhalation because of a retention prolonged beyond your limits, you should not worry. It only indicates that you must start again and reduce the length of retention. At first, you cannot stand much discomfort. With practice you will be able to increase the length of the retention until there is a struggle between your breath and yourself. Gradually extend the practice of breath retention until you feel a sensation of fatigue – not of suffocation – and until you begin to perspire. At that moment you feel a very special vibration: 'The student should

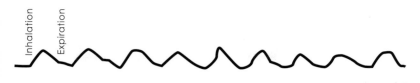

IRREGULAR AND SUPERFICIAL NORMAL BREATHING

Correct

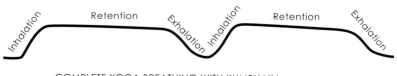

COMPLETE YOGA BREATHING WITH KUMBHAKA

Incorrect

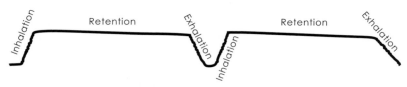

COMPLETE YOGA BREATHING WITH KUMNHAKA (SUDDEN CHGES, JERKY INHALATION AND EXHALATION TO BE AVOIDED)

practise Kumbhaka until he feels Prana penetrating the whole body, from head to toe. He should then exhale very slowly through the right nostril' (Hatha Yoga Pradipika, II,49). You should perform a cycle of five or six pranayamas with breath retention, then rest for a few minutes before starting another cycle. You will be surprised to find that breath retention is much easier during the second cycle than during the first. The reason is that breath retention strongly stimulates the spleen and makes it contract and expel large quantities of red corpuscles into the bloodstream. After a few deep breaths, the blood is enriched with red corpuscles and oxygen so that you can hold out longer and more easily. Do not time yourself. This typical Western propensity leads to a 'performance' which is not only opposed to the spirit of yoga but above all to the student's interest, since it incites him to go beyond his limits with all the dangers this involves. An occasional check is acceptable as an indication.

NOTE:
When you practise pranayama exercises with breath retention of more than ten seconds, it is indispensable to accompany them by Jalandhara Banda (see page 133).

15 | Anuloma Viloma

We have thus cleared the way to pranayama with Kumbhaka exercises. Yoga followers who have regularly practised the preparation exercises for pranayama can now begin breath retention. Of course the instructions concerning concentration, etc. still apply.

The exercise mentioned on page 69 (Section 12), should be performed with the following changes:

> Exhale through the left nostril;
> Inhale through the left nostril;
> Kumbhaka with full lungs;
> Exhale through the right nostril;
> Inhale through the right nostril;
> Kumbhaka with full lungs.

Repeat this cycle immediately.

During retention both nostrils are closed. Without Kumbhaka this exercise is known as Nadi Sodhana. The addition of breath retention modifies its nature and its name, which then becomes Anuloma Viloma, a very important and classical pranayama exercise.

1 6 | R h y t h m

The element we are now about to introduce into our pranayama exercises is of prime importance, the element of rhythm and of the proportions of the various phases of the act of breathing. The cosmos is full of rhythm. The rotation of the earth and its orbit around the sun regulate the alternation of day and night and of the seasons. These rhythms are not a matter of chance but the result of the inner structure of matter and of the universe. Rhythm is a fundamental phenomenon of the cosmos. In the course of evolution all life on earth, be it vegetable, animal or human, has been moulded by these rhythms. Is it mere coincidence that a lunar month and a woman's menstrual cycle are both twenty-eight days long? To go deeper into the effect of fundamental cosmic rhythms on the psycho-physiological behaviour of human beings would be beyond the scope of our study, but we do find that the human organism is very sensitive to rhythm and is impregnated with it. The most obvious and doubtless the most important rhythms are those of the heart and breathing, although cytology may have some surprises in store for us.

The interdependence of these biological rhythms comes from the very constitution of our organism. The strength and therefore the rhythm of our heartbeats are determined by the power of the heart muscle, by the viscosity of the blood and by the diameter of the blood vessels from the aorta to the capillaries, the latter so fine that the red corpuscles (five million of which barely fill a cubic millimetre) must creep through them one by one according to the requirements of the organism. Placed end to end the capillaries would be 100,000 kilometres long with a surface area of about 7,000 square metres. They constitute the real contact between the blood and the cells, immersed in the extracellular fluid. The circulation of the blood through the capillaries remains a mystery, but a well-known and a very simple physical law can help us to calculate the power required by a pump to circulate a known quantity of fluid of a certain viscosity at a given speed. By this calculation we find that the heart, in order to overcome the internal resistance of the capillaries to the progression of the blood, should be thousands of times more powerful than it actually is. That is why it is more and more commonly accepted that the heart confines itself to driving the blood into the arteries and arterioles and as far as the capillaries, which in turn guide it through their intricate net-work. So the heart may not be the actual motor of blood circulation in the capillaries any more than the stomach pushes food through the digestive tract; it is the intestine itself which, by its peristaltic mo-tion, moves the alimentary bolus. It is probably in a similar fashion that the capillaries drive the blood through their ultramicroscopic network. Just as the intestinal contractions depend upon the stomach and vice versa, the heart rhythm is closely related to the bloodflow in the capillaries, which corresponds to the fundamental rhythm of the organism. This bloodflow depends on our cell requirements. The cardiac rhythm is therefore an integral part of the physiological needs of the whole organism; the breathing and the heartbeats of a running man are increased and accelerated. Thus all the biological rhythms of our organism are integrated, so that their harmony signifies health while their discordance leads to sickness. The following excerpt from Dr Salmanoff's *Secrets et sagesse du corps is significant:*

'There are cases, not at all rare, in which a patient's death cannot be explained by the development of morbid phenomena, nor by the fail-ure of the great, basic functions (breathing, circulation, elimination), nor by a serious complication preceding death. One likely hypothesis remains: a break in the synchronisation of the biological rhythms.

'In a healthy individual the frequency of breathing should vary between 16 and 20 per minute, while the heart should contract from 72 to 80 times, and the kidneys filter urine at a definite rate. The lungs, heart, myoglobine, lactic acid and muscle fibres release oxygen to a definite rhythm: 300 times a minute. It is surprising to find a pre-estab-lished rate of roughly 1:4: 16 between these rhythms: breathing 18 per minute, heart contractions 72 per minute, myoglobin disassociation rhythm 300 times per minute...

'It requires one respiration to deliver sufficient oxygen for four contractions of the myocardium. It takes one contraction of the myocardium (heart muscle) to deliver sufficient oxygen for the four contractions of the fibrils of the striped and the smooth muscles. The synchronisation of rhythm between the frequency of breathing, the number of systolic contractions and the number of myoglobin deliver-ies to the muscular fibrils is obvious. The red corpuscles are the carriers of oxygen. If oxygen simply dissolved in the blood, not linked to the red corpuscles, the heart would have to beat forty times faster than it does in order to ensure the breathing of the tissues.

'Research into the rhythm of various physiological functions might provide most interesting data.

'The peristaltic rhythm of a full stomach and that of an empty stomach, the rhythm of secretion of the gastric and intestinal juices, of the liver and gall bladder bile, the length and rhythm of some metabolic reactions, might very well widen our knowledge of synchronised rhythms.'

Rhythm also has an effect on our endurance. We all know that we can cover considerable distances with little fatigue at a steady rhythm but we get tired quickly if our step is irregular or unrhythmic. The introduction of rhythm into work regulates it and reduces muscular and intellectual fatigue. Through dance and music rhythm becomes perceptible and alive, influencing the emotions and the mind itself. Eventually rhythm affects the whole human being, leaving no part untouched.

Yogis, with their sharp sense of observation, have not failed to notice these peculiarities. Thousands of years before Salmanoff they had noticed that four heartbeats corresponded to one breath. Therefore, the yogis' first objective, where rhythm is concerned, is to establish firmly the synchronisation of heartbeats with breathing. They also noticed that it was possible to affect all physiological and psychological functions of a human being by deliberately altering these fundamental rhythms. The rhythmic breathing exercises below must be placed in such a perspective.

Rhythmic breathing

In your favourite position for pranayama exercises, wait until your breathing acquires a normal resting rhythm while you concentrate on your heartbeats or your blood pulsations. This is not difficult: you need only concentrate on the heart region to become conscious of it at will. If you do not succeed, you can take your pulse at the wrist. When you feel the heartbeats clearly – with or without the help of the pulse – you synchronise the cardiac and respiratory rhythms consciously. Count two beats for inhaling, four for exhaling and breathe this way for about one minute: we already know that for pranayama exercises exhalation usually lasts twice as long as inhalation. This rhythm is indeed quite normal. When you have the opportunity, watch a purring cat: follow its breathing rhythm by looking at its belly and you will notice that exhalation lasts twice as long as inhalation. Gradually lengthen your breathing; count three beats for inhalation (*purak*) and six for exhalation (*rechak*). If you do so without discomfort or effort, increase to four beats for purak, eight for rechak, and so forth.

No mention has yet been made of breath retention. First of all it is essential to let the rhythm establish itself and then extend itself before introducing Kumbhaka, breath retention, which requires separate training (see p. 82). Perfect synchronisation will soon take place and you will notice that your mind becomes absorbed by regular, conscious and rhythmic breathing. This is one of the goals of the exercise. The result is peace and serenity, achieved by the magic of rhythm, the antidote to the excitement of modern life. There is nothing like rhythmic breathing to calm frayed nerves, to quiet minds disturbed by the tensions of our frantic civilisation.

All the exercises described in the preceding sections may be improved by the synchronisation of breathing and the heartbeats, particularly when practising alternate breathing. If we have not discussed rhythm earlier in this book it is because there are too many details at the beginning of these exercises, and to become preoccupied at this stage with a new factor would be a source of distraction rather than an element of integration. As soon as you have sufficiently assimilated the technique of alternate breathing you can and must bring rhythm into your pranayama exercises and so increase their efficacy. The duration of each breath has limited importance, but rhythm is the decisive element.

Complete rhythmic breathing
Before you practise alternate rhythmic breathing you should practise complete yoga breathing with control of the abdominal muscles and with short breath retention. Ratio: at the beginning, Puraka, one unit; Kumbhaka, two units. In other words, inhale for four beats, hold your breath for eight beats, then exhale for eight beats. By trial and error you fill find the optimum duration of a unit which will allow you to carry on almost indefinitely without fatigue. That essential, concentration, is helped by rhythm, which holds the attention. With practice you will lengthen your retention and reach the classical rhythm by successive stages: Puraka, one unit; Kumbhaka, four units; Rechaka, two units. Therefore, if inhalation corresponds to four heartbeats (one

unit), hold your breath with full lungs for sixteen beats (four units) and exhale for eight beats (two units).

Alternate rhythmic breathing

When you have become accustomed to the preceding exercise you can practise alternate breathing with breath retention at the same rhythm 1:4:2. This most classic and powerful exercise is harmless if you observe these basic conditions: ease, concentration, rhythm. Duration is a quite secondary element. I emphasise this point because Westerners often tend to consider duration as an objective. Not only is it the least important element but it is perhaps the only one which might have drawbacks. As long as you apply the rules for breath retention given in the previous section with all your exercises you will not run any risks. Practise with perseverance, regularity and smoothness until the rhythm is so deeply ingrained that you will no longer need to count. Then rhythmic breathing will be as natural as walking. In pranayama, more than in anything else, everything is linked, but be careful not to rush through any stages; they are all indispensable and must be followed one by one. In the end, not hurrying is the best way of going fast and safely.

1 7 | Viloma Pranayama

It is to be regretted that Viloma Pranayama is so little known in the West. Besides its own benefits it allows the practice of breath retention without danger. Its fundamental characteristic is to spread retention over several stages of either inhalation or exhalation.

Technique

Posture. As for other pranayama exercises, it may be performed either in a yoga posture or in a low chair. It may also be performed while walking, or even while lying down.

Cycle A: fractional inhalation. In this exercise rhythm plays an essential part. Before starting Viloma take your pulse and get accustomed to your heartbeat. At first keep your thumb on your pulse until you are fully conscious of this rhythm, which will act as a metronome. Then inhale through both nostrils for two heartbeats, hold your breath for two beats, inhale again for two beats, stop your breath again for two beats, etc., until your lungs are quite full. Then (complete yoga inhalation in three stages with control of the abdominal muscles) hold your breath again for from five to ten seconds, then slowly exhale through both nostrils. As soon as the lungs are empty, start another inhalation in the same way. A series of five complete inhalations, followed by a continuous exhalation forms cycle A of Viloma Pranayama.

Cycle B: fractional exhalation. In cycle B the exhalation is performed in successive stages: two beats for retention, two beats for exhalation, two beats for retention, two beats for exhalation, and so forth until the lungs are quite empty. After a brief retention, from five to ten seconds, inhale without any interruption. Five such breaths make up cycle B. One cycle A plus one cycle B make a complete Viloma Pranayama. Then rest in Shavasana, breathing normally. Experienced students may start another complete cycle provided they do not feel tired. Pranayama must be stopped at once as soon as there is a feeling of fatigue or discomfort. Concentration and rhythm, rather than duration, are the essential elements of this exercise.

Improving the exercise

Improvement does not consist of increasing the duration, which will always remain two heartbeats, but the number of stages. To increase the number it is necessary to decrease the amount of air exhaled (or inhaled) at each stage. With beginners the lungs will be filled (or emptied) in three or four stages only. With practice it is possible to decrease the amount of air exhaled (or inhaled) to reach eight, ten or more stages. In Viloma Pranayama breathing is always silent; each stop must be gentle and the glottis must be closed.

Viloma Pranayama with Mula Bandha

Viloma Pranayama accompanied with Mula Bandha becomes a real pranayama exercise in every sense. During the training period the yoga student concentrates on the process itself and on maintaining the rhythm. As soon as the exercise has become familiar - after a few days' practice - it should be supplemented by Mula Bandha. This is a contraction of the anal sphincter and of the muscle which raises the anus. The result is a contraction of the whole perineum (see p. 194). Mula Bandha accompanies each retention. Therefore you must contract the anus at each stage of breath retention. Whenever you inhale or exhale, whether it is cycle A or cycle B, you release Mula Bandha. During Mula Bandha you should concentrate on Muladhara, the contracted anal area. Thus Mula Bandha occurs at each stage of retention and also during the five to ten seconds retention period which ends inhalation or exhalation.

Advantages

This exercise has all the beneficial effects of pranayama with breath retention while being absolutely harmless. Only people with heart trouble should refrain from it as indeed from all pranayama exercises with retention (see counter-indications mentioned earlier).

In pranayama exercises with continuous retention, we sometimes go unintentionally beyond our capabilities. During retention we may think we can hold the breath comfortably for a few more seconds, but when we must exhale as prescribed – exhalation lasting twice as long as inhalation – things go wrong: we are forced to exhale too fast. The exercise is thus distorted and its rhythm and proportions destroyed. In Viloma Pranayama retentions are brief; the exercise is easily controlled and is automatically regulated since only the number of stages varies. Viloma Pranayama helps to concentrate and so puts rhythm into breathing. Inhaling for two seconds, then holding your breath (with Mula Bandha) for two seconds (or four heartbeats, which is more rational) forces you to concentrate on the exercise and prevents you from being distracted.

This exercise constitutes a smooth, gradual and imperceptible training for pranayama. The air cells open harmoniously and gently; breathing is slowed down and the gas exchange in the lungs takes place under optimum conditions. Viloma Pranayama does not harm the lungs. The yoga student is warned when he comes near his limitations and does not run the risk of exceeding them inadvertently. It is the ideal exercise for those who practise pranayama without an experienced guide. This exercise offers all the advantages described in the previous sections, those gained from pranayama with retention and those from pranayama with Mula Bandha. It has the special advantage of normalising blood pressure. People who suffer from a slightly high or low blood pressure will find the condition gradually improved.

Another improvement
During fractional inhalation (or between two stages of retention) imagine that you are smelling the fragrance of a rose while concentrating on the stream of fresh air which should be felt high up in the nasal cavities. These are covered with extremely sensitive nerve endings and are the main organs for the absorption of atmospheric prana. This mental image helps your mind to focus on your respiration. That is why sticks of sandalwood are burned in India. They perfume and purify the air while leading to improved concentration.

In bed
This exercise may be performed lying down, for instance in bed at night before falling asleep, or in the morning before getting up. At night choose cycle B, which is sedative and induces deep sleep. In the morning, cycle A is better to 'pep you up' and to dispel the last mists of sleepiness. If the exercise is performed lying down during the day, five A cycles should be followed by five B cycles. During the day, however, it is preferable to practise while seated.

Viloma Pranayama while walking
Viloma Pranayama can easily be performed while walking in the open

air. As with other exercises of rhythmic breathing, the step may be used as a metronome. On flat ground you can find your rhythm quite easily, but the rhythm must be readjusted constantly if the ground is uneven and the step irregular.

With Viloma Pranayama the number of stages can vary at will and the exercise can be adapted to the breathing capacity of the student and to his walking pace. Also when walking the breath retention which normally takes place at the end of exhalation (or inhalation) is omitted: inhale for two steps, hold the breath for two steps, inhale again for two steps, hold the breath again and so forth until the lungs are full. The lungs are then emptied slowly but without stopping, and the process is started again as described above. Do five A cycles (during inhalation) followed by five B cycles (during exhalation), then rest, letting the breath come and go spontaneously without worrying about rhythm. As soon as the breathing is back to normal the exercise may be resumed.

There is another difference: Mula Bandha is optional.

Viloma Pranayama while walking is a remarkable tonic. Try it for a few minutes: you will find some warmth in your cheeks and in your whole body, a sign that cell breathing – the true internal breathing – is stimulated. You may, if you wish, imagine the 'OM' which accompanies each inhalation or exhalation. Never try to increase the number of stages: the exercise must always remain easy and comfortable; it must not cause any pressure. This is the guarantee of safety.

18 | Prana Mudra or Shanti Mudra

Through the centuries yoga has been transmitted orally from master to disciple under the seal of secrecy. In ancient scriptures the secret was protected by the brevity of the texts or by the occult nature and the ambiguity of the formulations: 'Like a most precious jewel, this exercise must remain secret.' For the most part these texts cannot be used without an intelligent commentary. For instance, we find in Gheranda Samhita, Chapters 1, 16, 17 and 18, the following description of Varisara Dhauti, which corresponds to Shanka Prakshalana:

'Fill the mouth with water as far back as the throat, then swallow it slowly; make it go through the stomach, push it downwards and expel it through the rectum. This process must remain most secret. It cleanses the body. If it is carefully practised the disciple will acquire a bright body [that is, purified clean (translator's note)]. Varisara is the highest Dhauti. Whoever practises it with ease cleanses his foul body and transforms it into a pure body.'

Quite certainly nobody could perform this exercise with the help of these instructions alone, other than the limited circle of initiates. Yet it is emphasised that the process must 'remain most secret'. We read on (I, 21): 'This form of Dhauti [Agnisara Dhauti] must be kept very secret'; (I, 22): 'This Dhauti must remain a great secret and must not be revealed to anyone.' This anxiety, bordering on obsession, to preserve the secret which pervades yoga literature shocks many Westerners. They see in it an expression of egoism on the part of the great rishis who deliberately deprive humanity of their valuable knowledge. The initiates reply that the rishis did not impose this rule of secrecy, that the instruction was not given to deprive foreigners of the fruit of the rishis' experiments but to protect them from some dangers. The rishis add that anyone who really wishes to practise yoga will find his master. But this is only a partial explanation. The rule of secrecy derives from the very principle of transmitting yoga on an individual basis, whereby the master initiates and guides the student step by step. That is why today, in many Indian ashrams, students who have the same master are still not allowed to communicate to each other the exercises they have learned. This prohibition leaves the master free to reveal to each disciple individually and at the right time the techniques which correspond to his stage of development. It enables him to personalise his teachings and even to contradict himself occasionally. Actually, these contradictions are only apparent, as an exercise may be right for one disciple and wrong for another. It is therefore logical to forbid the swapping of techniques. Yoga students accept and respect this willingly because they have complete trust in their masters. Besides, shared secrecy creates a very special bond; secret societies derive much of their power from it. Some esoteric orders preserve many practices which could be revealed to the public at large without any problem, but restricting these rites and practices to the initiated maintains their value. Often, too, secrecy is a protection against hostility and a means of withstanding the test of time. Finally, noncommunication protects against changes of nature; for when knowledge is diffused without restriction it escapes all control and opens the way to all sorts of distortions. The student himself benefits from secret practice because it shields him from curiosity and gives him increased strength, since it discourages him from substituting words for deeds. He who talks to everyone about his plans seldom carries them out. Be discreet about your practice; do not broadcast that you are doing yoga, especially during the first months. I believe that many beginners have not persevered solely because they talked about it too much. Men of action spare their words!

So there are quite a few justifications for secrecy. Yet the spread of yoga all over the world seems to have put an end to that occult period. In fact, however, this is not the case. The orthodox in India are still hostile to any uncontrolled dissemination of yoga. To my knowledge the exercise described in this section has never before been published. Should we conclude that by divulging it I am violating the law of secrecy? I think not. In fact it is prescribed that 'this exercise must be performed in private, away from the presence of any witness'. Which is rather different. The exercise itself does not need to remain unknown to students, but its practice should be secret. It is possible to practise asanas in another's presence without noticeably diminishing their efficacy. But with Prana Mudra any other presence, even that of a friend experienced in yoga, constitutes a disturbing factor jeopardising its success.

Prana Mudra is a complete pranayama. Apart from its pranic aspect, its control of the body's 'spiritual' forces, it also belongs to the category of mudras or symbolic gestures, i.e. corporal expressions with a psychic resonance. This exercise needs to be studied with even greater care than the asanas, and every indication must be scrupulously followed.

Technique

Starting posture. Normally, this position should be the lotus exclusively. However, for Westerners who have not yet mastered padmasana, siddhasana, or even vajrasana, is acceptable. As an ultimate concession, and purely temporary, the exercise may be performed sitting on a chair, the hands on top of one another in the lap with palms upwards. The spine must be very straight.

The exercise

Before giving a detailed description, I advise the student to glance at the photographs and acquire a general idea of the movements.

This is a pranayama combined with arm and hand movements. First let us see what Prana Mudra looks like. During inhalation, which is slow and easy, the hands move from the lap and rise as the lungs fill; the arms are spread open when the lungs are full; after breath retention with full lungs, the hands slowly return to their starting position in the lap at the end of exhalation.

For each phase the details must be followed scrupulously. Do not hurry. Follow the instructions carefully, for each has a profound reason. You will be amply rewarded by the increased benefits from subsequent practice.

First step (starting with empty lungs). The exercise starts at the end of a complete exhalation, after contracting the abdominal muscles and expelling the last traces of air. This contraction is accompanied by Mula Bandha, a contraction of the anus. With empty lungs, pause for a few seconds to concentrate before starting on Prana Mudra. So long as inhalation has not yet started hands must remain motionless in the lap, palms upwards, fingers slightly bent. You are now ready for the second step.

Second step (beginning of inhalation). Diaphragmatic phase: slightly ease the contraction of the abdominal muscles and relax Mula Bandha.

Inhalation starts gently; while the air slowly enters both nostrils, the lowering of the diaphragm causes a slight pressure in the lower abdomen, the hands move from the lap, the elbows leave the body and the extended fingers point straight at the abdomen as if they were irradiating it. As the abdominal phase of the inhalation develops, the hands move up along and in front of the abdomen; they follow the ascent of the intra-abdominal pressure.

Third step. Costal phase: at the end of the abdominal phase the hands, with fingers extended, are still pointed towards the abdomen, level with the stomach and the solar plexus, opposite Manipura Chakra. Inhalation continues with the expansion of the thorax and the spreading of the ribs. While the upper lungs are filling up the hands continue their slow ascent and the elbows move away from the trunk; the chest expands harmoniously. The fingers, instead of pointing at the body, now move parallel to the thorax in front of the chest, rising until the end of the thoracic phase. A that point they are level with the collarbones, the elbows are far apart from the body and the arms are parallel with the ground.

Fourth step. Clavicular phase: the diaphragm has flattened out, the thorax has expanded but it is still possible to inhale a certain amount of air by raising the rib-cage under the collar-bones (see *Yoga Self-Taught*). With the completion of inhalation the hands pass in front of the throat and face and move away from the body until the arms are wide apart, with the palms turned upwards and forward as if to capture the rays of the rising sun. In the final posture the arms are extended from the shoulders and parallel to the ground. The muscles are relaxed and the lungs are full.

Fifth step (retention with full lungs). The student remains motionless in this receptive attitude and holds his breath as long as he comfortably can. This phase is fundamental. We shall return to it when we deal with concentration. During retention the student should naturally observe all the recommendations made earlier: comfort, ease, progressiveness.

Sixth step (exhalation). When retention ceases to be comfortable the student inhales a little fresh air, then lets exhalation begin in reverse order, which is contrary to the normal yoga exhalation. The top of the lungs empties first, which is easier when the elbows are drawn together at the beginning of the exhalation. The thorax then lowers itself and the abdomen flattens out. During exhalation the hands gradually come down and at the end they are replaced in the lap while the final abdominal contraction expels the last traces of air. Mula Bandha follows and the same process starts anew at once.

Concentration (during inhalation). *Abdominal phase:* concentrate on all parts of the abdomen as the fingers pass in front of them. Imagine that a pranic current exudes from the fingertips, radiates through all the organs and pervades them with consciousness and vitality. Concentrate especially when the hands pass in front of the solar plexus but without pausing. *Costal phase:* while the hands move in front of the thorax, visualise the air which enters and fills the lungs. *Clavicular phase:* concentrate on the warmth of your hands on your throat and face; radiate prana through the neck and the eyes.

Concentration (during retention). The essential phase of Prana Mudra takes place during breath retention when the arms are spread wide with the palms turned upwards towards the rising sun (whether real or imaginary is unimportant). This is based on the yoga concept of interaction of body and mind. Humanity did not wait for yogis or for modern psychology to find out that every psychic attitude is expressed outwardly in a body attitude, that every emotion has its physical expression. It is also true of animals: a dog expresses its pleasure by wagging its tail, while with cats, on the other hand, motion of the tail expresses excitement or annoyance. In human beings speech replaces movement, but movement remains a powerful means of expression. The intensity of expression in miming is often greater than that of an actor speaking.

Although it is a well-known fact that the body conveys moods through its movements and attitudes, the opposite – a physical attitude inducing a psychological state – is less commonly accepted and applied. Hufeland used to advise depressed persons to sit in front of a mirror and smile, for a feeling corresponding to the physical expression soon pervades the psyche. So it is on the principle of the reversible interaction of body upon the psyche that this part of the exercise is based. The welcoming gesture that marks the end of the exercise during retention is a sign of acceptance, of opening up to the universe.

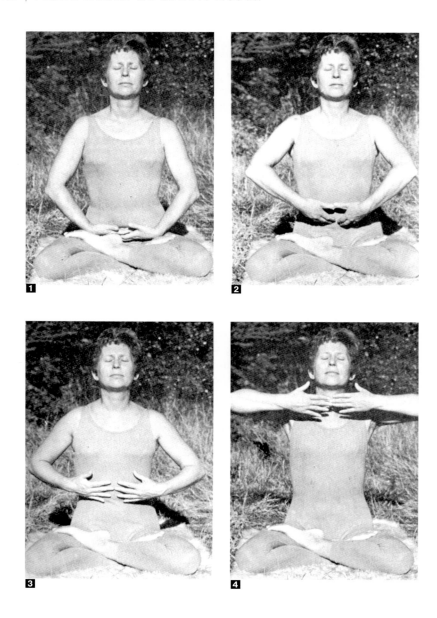

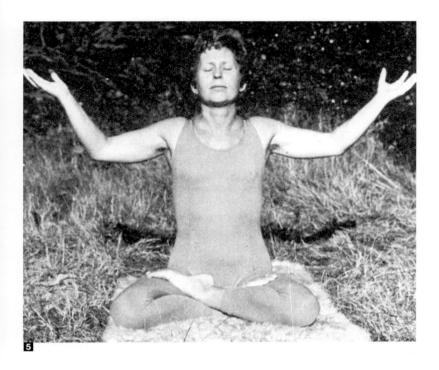

5

---

1 Start: in Lotus posture place your hands on your lap, palms upwards and with no stiffness in the arms. Relax the face muscles, look towards the tip of your nose without strain. Empty the lungs thoroughly by contracting the abdominal muscles. Mula Bandha.

2 *Beginning of inhalation, abdominal phase.* Direct the fingertips towards the lower abdomen, move the elbows away from the body, release the abdominal muscles. Stop Mula Bandha and let the air slowly enter the lungs. As the diaphragm descends, the hands continue their ascent towards the solar plexus. They will reach this level at the end of the abdominal phase

3 At the start of the thoracic phase spread the elbows to facilitate the expansion of the chest. The fingers flatten out, moving parallel with the ribs. The hands keep rising as the lungs fill up. When the expansion of the chest is nearly finished your hands are level with the collarbones.

4 Then the clavicular phase begins. At that point your hands pass in front of your throat and face.

5 Finally you reach the position represented on this picture after the lungs are entirely full of air. Hold your breath and let the mental attitude corresponding to this posture permeate your mind. Exhale and go back to your starting position in reverse order.

While the student listens to the psychic echo of the Mudra, holding his breath and with eyes closed, he visualises the rising sun, absorbs its radiance, lets the vitality of the cosmos pervade him. Yet this should not become an intellectual exercise; the mental attitude should come spontaneously. A wonderful relaxation then spreads through body and mind.

The chin is pointed upwards and directed towards the sun (real or imaginary). The muscles of the neck and arms stay relaxed. There is no stiffness in the wrists or fingers. This 'psychic climate', sometimes experienced during the first retention, becomes stronger with every retention. That is why Prana Mudra should be performed at least five times in succession.

Concentration during exhalation. During exhalation, concentrate on the slow and complete evacuation of the air from the lungs; think of every part of the body in front of which your hands are moving.

'OM'

The exercise is accompanied by Pranava or silent OM. During inhalation, the student listens to a long O… M… vibrating within him. During breath retention he may either keep absolute inner silence (without OM) and accept only a visualisation of the sun, or he may pronounce inwardly: 'shanti, shanti, shanti'.* During exhalation, listen to the inner OM. At the beginning, when learning the exercise, it will probably be impossible for the student to perform the movements, to concentrate on the various parts of his body and to listen to the OM as well! With practice, it can easily be done.

First, the arm movement must be correctly assimilated. It must flow gracefully without any stiffness or jerkiness. At the beginning it is helpful to practise in front of a mirror to check the movement and make sure that it is graceful: this is very important. A jerky movement affects the mental state. The various phases of the exercise must be linked. When the movement has been absorbed, concentrate on the various parts of your body and think about prana radiating through your fingers. Add OM at the very last.

Beneficial effects

* *Shanti* means Peace. It is better to use the Sanskrit expression, dragging out the Shan…followed by the syllable 'ti': Shan – ti!

To appreciate the efficacy of this exercise, it should be performed several times; immediately afterwards take a normal breath, remaining immobile, without moving your arms, your hands in your lap. You will notice at once how much more harmonious, how much deeper and happier inhalation is with Prana Mudra. You are more aware of the respiratory act, your mind can concentrate better. A sense of peace and serenity prevails during breath retention.

This exercise must be performed privately as the presence of a witness would be disturbing, particularly in the last phase when the relaxed face expresses inner emotion and shares in that serenity. It is even more unthinkable to perform this exercise in public as it might appear ridiculous to the uninitiated who would not understand its significance. The sages were right when they prescribed the secret practice of this exercise. Do not talk about it to anybody, do not cofide in any other student, not even in your spouse! Prana Mudra must remain private, lest it should lose part of its efficacy. The only authorised public practice is for training purposes, as for example in a class. Even then, you will soon notice that practising in company does not allow you to reach the required emotional intensity. Only a true master could, by this presence, release the emotional content of Prana Mudra in several students simultaneously.

19 | Control of the Abdomen

Despite their multiplicity, asanas rely on a limited number of basic principles: immobility, breath control, effortlessness, muscle stretching and mental concentration. Ignoring or misunderstanding a single one of these factors will impair the efficacy of the postures. The same is true of pranayama and yogic breathing, one of the main supports of which is the active behaviour of the abdominal wall, affecting the respiratory process and determining its effectiveness.

Control of the abdominal muscles enables yogis to modify pressure in the abdomen and thorax at will, with important repercussions. It is therefore regrettable, to say the least, that Western students should be left in total ignorance of the subject. In Western countries the technique of complete yogic breathing is well known, but precise and complete instructions concerning the highly active role of the abdominal wall are practically non-existant. They are all the more necessary as yoga techniques for pranayama differ from our Western concept, according to which the abdominal muscles must remain passive and relaxed during the whole respiratory act. By yielding without any resistance to the pressure exerted by the diaphragm on the viscera the abdominal muscles permit abdominal breathing which, as its name implies, is accompanied by a dilation of the abdomen.

I believe that the Western idea of abdominal breathing with relaxed muscles came about as a reaction against the 'gymnastic' technique of breathing, which is almost entirely costal. The two drawings below, taken from a book on respiratory rehabilitation, are quite revealing. The author of the work in question, who shall remain nameless, rightly condemns 'gymnastic' breathing, which simply omits abdominal breathing: he replaces it with abdominal breathing, which allows a fuller and easier inhalation. But abdominal breathing has several drawbacks for the practice of pranayama. Because of the influence of such writings and the lack of precise guidance, this concept of the role of the abdominal muscles has spread to a number of yoga disciples who think they must relax them and allow the abdomen to become distended during inhalation. It is mostly men who breathe that way, for women refrain out of vanity (to keep their 'figures'); they are very reluctant when it comes to distending the abdominal muscles lest they develop

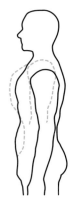
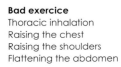
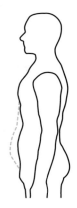

Bad exercice
Thoracic inhalation
Raising the chest
Raising the shoulders
Flattening the abdomen

Good exercice
Abdominal inhalation
Immobilisation of the chest
Immobilisation of the shoulders
Expansion of the abdomen during
inhalation

These drawings show that diaphragmatic breathing was substituted for thoracic breathing, probably an improvement but not enough.

paunches. No criticism is intended by the use of inverted commas with the word 'figures', for the female concern for them is closer to reality than is the case with those gentlemen who let their abdominal muscles become flabby. Incidentally, it might be as well to use the expression 'diaphragmatic phase' instead of 'abdominal phase' from now on.

True, the diaphragmatic phase of yogic breathing is the most important; it is not only possible but indispensable to control the abdominal muscles when performing it. Pranayama without active control of the abdominal muscles is nonsense.

To understand what goes on mechanically, we shall compare the trunk to a cylinder divided into compartments, rigid at the thoracic level, flexible at the abdominal level (that flexibility depends very much on the tonus of the abdominal muscles). As the abdominal wall is flexible and can be controlled by willpower, its behaviour influences all breathing processes. Imagine a piston (the diaphragm) moving up and down inside the cylinder. It is surprising that the very existence of the diaphragm is so little known; very few are aware of its exact shape, of its position and of the amplitude of its motion. According to Dr A. Salmanoff, even part of the medical profession underestimates its importance:

'The story of the physiopathology of the diaphragm is both funny and sad. Of course diaphragmatic pleurisy or paralysis and subphrenic abscesses are clinically well known. The diaphragm is casually described as a fairly unimportant muscle which plays a great part in respiration... The physiopathological role of the diaphragm in the evolution of chronic diseases is completely ignored and neglected in medical literature...

'Let us take a close look at the diaphragm and try to assess its activity in relation to the various functions of our organism. In a healthy body the diaphragm moves up and down 18 times per minute; it travels 4 centimetres up and 4 centimetres down. The amplitude of these movements is approximately 8 centimetres. 19 movements per minute or 1,000 an hour and 24,000 in 24 hours! Just think for a moment about the amount of work produced by this muscle whose surface area is considerable. It is the most powerful muscle in our body; it acts like a perfect force-pump, compressing the liver, the spleen, the intestines, and stimulating the whole abdominal and portal circulation.

'By compressing all the lymphatic and blood vessels of the abdomen, the diaphragm aids the veinous circulation from the abdomen towards the thorax.

'The number of movements of the diaphragm per minute is a quarter of those of the heart. But its haemodynamic power is much greater than that of the cardiac contractions because the surface of the force-pump is much greater and because its propelling power is superior to that of the heart. We have only to visualise the surface of the diaphragm to accept the fact that it acts like another heart.

'Laboratory physiologists should start giving us a true account of the diaphragmatic blood flow compared with the cardiac flow; also of the role of the diaphragm in 'cleaning out' the liver and spleen blood reservoirs. (These may, under certain conditions - during the cold season for instance - hold thirty to fifty per cent of the volume of circulating blood.) They should explain the role of the diaphragmatic pump in propelling the lymph towards the thoracic canal; also the role

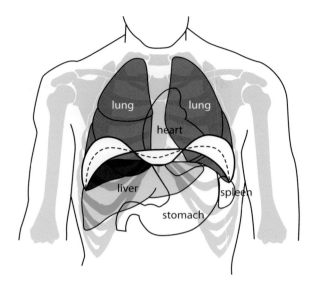

of the diaphragm in the systematic compression (24,000 times a day) of the intestinal village: – the sole seat of general metabolism – where the mysterious transformation of assimilable, nutritious substances intended for the tissues and cells takes place. The dia-phragm is like a good, willing mill, working for the nourishment of the organism.

'By compressing the liver systematically, the diaphragm facilitates and may even direct the flow of bile, ensures the blood circulation of the liver and acts indirectly on the various functions of the liver. If we remember the role of the diaphragm in the whole hepatic physiology, we shall easily understand the relative value of the various functional explorations of the liver since, unfortunately, we accept as decisive the results of tests made on an isolated liver which exists only in the imagination of laboratory workers.

'By improving the function of the diaphragm we shall always im-prove the functions of the liver, even if the tests are catastrophic.'

Clearly, the diaphragm can play its full role only if diaphragmatic breathing includes control of the abdominal muscles. Let us first examine what happens during the diaphragmatic phase with relaxed abdominal muscles, then compare with what occurs when they are controlled. The drawing below illustrates the difference.

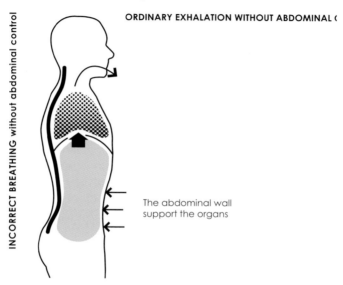

INCORRECT BREATHING without abdominal control

ORDINARY EXHALATION WITHOUT ABDOMINAL (

The abdominal wall support the organs

A. *Exhalation without abdominal control.* The diaphragm is high. The abdominal muscles simply follow the exhalation, holding the visceral mass. There is no forced exhalation. The abdominal cavity has become egg-shaped. The viscera are not subject to any noticeable compression since the abdominal wall is not taut.

B. *Situation at the end of inhalation without abdominal control.* After the diaphragmatic inhalation *without* abdominal control, the diaphragm has moved down and the lower lungs have filled with air. The objective has been reached: to inhale the maximum volume of air into the lower lungs by lowering and flattening the diaphragm. We notice that the abdominal cavity, which was egg-shaped at the start, now has the shape of a flattened balloon, but its volume is practically unchanged: the organs have simply moved down and forward.

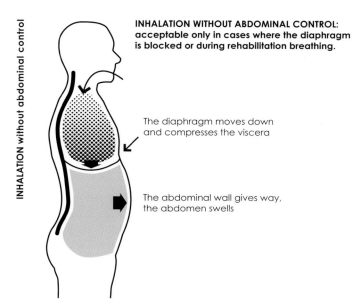

INHALATION without abdominal control

INHALATION WITHOUT ABDOMINAL CONTROL: acceptable only in cases where the diaphragm is blocked or during rehabilitation breathing.

The diaphragm moves down and compresses the viscera

The abdominal wall gives way, the abdomen swells

In the long run, a permanent deformation of the abdominal wall and belly may result. Breathing becomes more and more abdominal with consequent disadvantages which will be described later. Gorged with an abnormal quantity of blood, the organs become congested, blood circulation and biological processes are slowed down. Normally discouraged, this way of breathing is inadmissible in pranayama as, besides other disadvantages, it hinders thoracic and clavicular breathing. The following two diagrams illustrate the correct way of breathing: with abdominal control.

C Full exhalation with abdominal control. At the end of exhalation, the contracted abdominal muscles (which were not relaxed during inhalation) push the viscera backwards and upwards, and help the ascent of the diaphragmatic piston, thus permitting the expulsion of maximum residual air. The inner abdominal and thoracic pressures increase. The compressed sponge-like organs, having disgorged the excess of blood, resume their normal shape and volume.

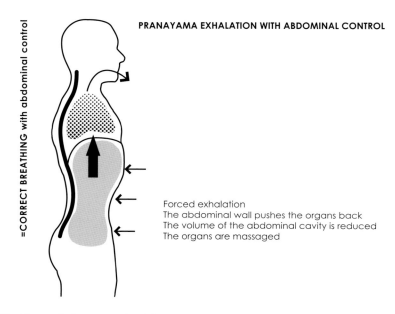

=CORRECT BREATHING with abdominal control

PRANAYAMA EXHALATION WITH ABDOMINAL CONTROL

Forced exhalation
The abdominal wall pushes the organs back
The volume of the abdominal cavity is reduced
The organs are massaged

D. *Yoga inhalation with abdominal control.* During inhalation the pis-ton-like diaphragm gradually comes down; at the end of inhalation it is as low as in breathing without abdominal control (illustration B). There is no reduction in the inhaled volume of air, although, during the lowering of the diaphragm, the abdominal muscles resist instead of yielding softly to the visceral mass pushed back by the diaphragm.

PRANAYAMA INHALATION WITH ABDOMINAL CONTROL

CORRECT BREATHING with abdominal control

Pressure from the diaphragm pushes the viscera back but the firm counter-pressure from the abdominal muscles, while it does not decrease the volume of air inhaled, increases the inner abdominal pressure.

Under the navel the abdominal muscles remain contracted (but not stiff). Above the navel they yield slightly without ceasing to control the pressure from the organs. It follows that in positions C and D the volume of the abdominal cavity is smaller than in A and B. The abdomen is not distorted: *this volume (C and D) is the ideal one*. Owing to their spongy nature, these organs return to their normal shape and form as soon as they empty themselves. Moreover, the antagonism (indicated by arrows) between the pressure from the diaphragm and the resistance of the abdominal wall increases the inner abdominal pressure. As a result, the viscera are massaged and strongly invigorated. All physiological functions are stimulated. Besides, only abdominal inhalation (which results in an intensification of abdominal control) allows a correct performance of the thoracic *and clavicular area*.

The three phases of complete yogic breathing can only be achieved successfully if they are performed within constant abdominal control. This is the only way of breathing which gives pranayama all its good effects and all its significance. Diaphragmatic inhalation with abdominal control keeps the abdominal and thoracic phases balanced.

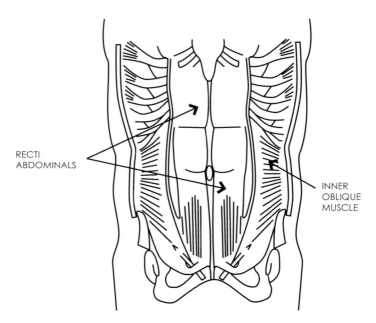

RECTI ABDOMINALS

INNER OBLIQUE MUSCLE

Physiological repercussions

The *active* role of the abdominal muscles has been little mentioned except in *Yoga Mimansa* by Shrimat Kuvalayananda, founder of the Institute of Scientific Research on Yoga at Lonavla, in a booklet published in 1930 and now out of print. Here is a translation of the fundamental excerpt:

'In pranayama, the study of pressure mochfications has great importance in the understanchng of the physiology of yoga exercises which are orientated toward spiritual fulfilment. Yoga processes for awakening Kundalini are mostly characterised by two factors. They involve either the elongation of the spine and its annexes, or the peculiarity of attracting a large quantity of blood to the tissues around the spine, especially in the pelvic and lumbar regions. In pranayama with abdominal control, stretching the spine is achieved by working on the contracted diaphragm, in particular through the action of its two.* At

---

* Crura is the plural of 'crus' which designates the two fibrous prolongations of the diaphragmatic dome linked to the lumbar vertebrae. They are truly the pillars of diaphragm.

the completion of the deepest possible inhalation, when the diaphragm is as contracted and as low as possible, it is pushed upwards by the large straight muscles (in the centre of the abdomen) which compress the viscera. That force is opposed by the contracted diaphragm and its two crura. In this manner a continuous traction is exerted on the spine and its adjacent parts. We can see that the high intra-abdominal pressure created in pranayama by the action and reaction of the anatomical parts as well as by the upward traction of the two crura is responsible for the awakening of Kundalini.'

The *difference of pressure* in the trunk – that is, between the abdomen and the surrounding air in the thorax and in the lungs – is considerably accentuated when the abdominal wall remains controlled and contracted. The struggle between the diaphragm, which is going down, and the abdominal muscles, which are resisting, has a direct effect on the abdominal organs but none on the thorax.

To sum up: at the abdominal level, higher pressure; at the thoracic level, depression during inhalation (otherwise the outside air could not enter the lungs). That difference between the increased positive pres-sure in the abdomen and the normal depression of the thorax has very important consequences for the circulation of the blood.

The two levels are separated by the diaphragmatic 'vault'. It is crossed by some blood vessels, in particular by the lower vena cava which collects the venous blood from the sub-diaphragmatic level of the body, that is to say, from all the abdominal viscera. It is through the lower vena cava that the intra-abdominal pressure finds its outlet. If compressing a balloon filled with liquid, the inside pressure increases. If the balloon has an opening fitted with a pipe facing upwards, the pressure will cause the liquid to rise. The abdomen behaves like that balloon, the lower vena cava serving as a pipe. The pressure exerted on the abdominal viscera by the struggle between diaphragm and abdominal muscles propels the venous blood from the viscera at the subdiaphragmatic level toward the thoracic level.

Instead of stagnating in the viscera, the venous blood shoots through the diaphragm toward the heart, which sends it to the lungs, where it gets rid of excess CO_2 and is replenished with oxygen and prana. It is as if the thorax literally sucked in the blood from the lower level. That suction is proportional to the difference of pressure between the levels. Breathing with abdominal control considerably accelerates the circulation of the venous blood in the abdomen and, in fact, in the whole system. Thanks to this powerful stimulus masses of stagnating blood are recycled, purified in the lungs and reinjected into the general circulatory system: they are going to revitalise the whole organism.

Back to the heart. Since half the population of industrialised countries are unfortunately threatened with cardiovascular ailments (heart attacks, etc.) it may be thought that this kind of breathing would be dangerous to such people. But this is not so: the lowering of the diaphragm relieves the heart, which is not compressed at any time, and the stimulation of venous circulation lightens its task. That is why doctors attached to the Lonavla laboratory declare: 'Pranayama is one of the best exercises for delicate hearts and weak lungs. Pranayama gives wonderful results when its physiology is understood and applied correctly.' However I emphasise that persons with weak hearts or delicate lungs must be very careful concerning breath retention.[*]

Contra-indications of Kumbhaka
It might be objected, however, that if the high pressure in the abdomen sends venous blood upwards through the lower vena cava, the same high pressure should curb the flow of arterial blood which descends into the abdomen through the abdominal aorta to feed the whole sub-diaphragmatic level of the body. The two effects should cancel each other out, but in fact do not. There are two reasons: as blood circulates in a closed circuit any acceleration of the blood flow at any point of the circuit accelerates the circulation in the whole network.[**] The intra-abdominal high pressure does not 'flatten' the aorta, since the arterial walls are rigid enough to resist such an increase of pressure mechanically. The heart does not have to make a greater effort to propel the blood towards the lower part of the compressed abdomen since the arterial blood is more or less drawn into the organs after the venous blood has been pushed upwards. Thus the heart works under the best possible conditions.

Should there still be any doubt, the following passages by Lonavla research workers should remove it:

_____

[*] See Section 14 p.82

[**] The reverse is just as true. Even the slightest interference with the circulation by compression must be avoided (e.g. narrow shoes, belts, collars, or even tight rings).

'Two positions have been prescribed for inhalation. Western respiratory physical culture recommends that the abdominal muscles be relaxed and distended by the pressure of the viscera pushed forward and downwards. Contrary to this, *yoga techniques* demand that these muscles remain contracted.

'Western medical authorities claim that the distended abdomen enables the diaphragm to move further down, which would provide a larger thoracic capacity and therefore a greater volume of inhaled air. According to them, controlling the abdominal wall would slow down the descent of the diaphragm, would limit the expansion of the thorax and therefore reduce the absorption of air. We have made a number of experiments in this field and have found this Western assertion to be more imaginary than real.* Our experiments lead us to conclude that the fall in intrapulmonary pressure is greater when inhaling with abdominal control than with relaxed abdominal muscles, and that the lung capacity increases considerably when inhaling with abdominal control, much more so than with a relaxed and distended abdomen.

Yoga practice

The importance of abdominal control became most clearly apparent to me while practising under a Yoga master in South India. During pranayama I saw the master controlling that tension by pressing his thumbs against the abdominal wall above the pubic symphysis, at the point of insertion of the large straight muscles, to make sure that it was correct (see photograph).

When controlling the abdominal wall during each phase of breathing (inhalation – exhalation – retention), the increase of pressure in the trunk is very noticeable. After breathing thus for one or two minutes it is normal at first to feel some fatigue in the abdominal and intercostal muscles. However, a sensation of general euphoria is experienced. A pleasant warmth, first felt in the cheeks, spreads to the whole body, indicating that cellular breathing has been stimulated.

I am convinced that the lungs hold both oxygen and prana better when intra-abdominal pressure is strong. Besides, the contraction of the abdomen during exhalation, especially at its end, draws the residual air out of the lungs much better. After a short adjustment period,

---

* I have visited the Lonavla laboratory: its equipment is up to the standards of a Western laboratory and its scientific staff carries out the experiments as rigorously as could be desired.

which varies according to the intensity of practice and the quality of the respiratory muscles of the individual, people do not wish to practise differently.

How to learn by yourself
Active control of the abdomen applies to all phases of pranayama but it is particularly indispensable during breath retention with full lungs. Before teaching yourself the correct abdominal muscle control, it is useful to examine the abdominal wall more closely. It is made up of several layers of muscles, some placed obliquely, others horizontally or vertically. The rectii abodominis, muscles which extend from the pubis to the thorax (sternum and ribs), are among the most important. They play the principal part in controlling breathing. The area between the naval and the point of the sternum is far less resistant than the area below the navel. To verify this, hold your breath with full lungs, stiffen the abdominal wall, then hit the area below the navel with the side of the palm: it can withstand even violent blows painlessly. Above the navel a much lighter blow will be painful.

And now to practice: sit down in lotus, siddhasana or vajrasana. Straighten your spine by stretching the back muscles and tilt the pelvis forward a little. The loins should be slightly arched. In order to acquire the correct lotus position automatically, just make sure both knees touch the ground since, in so doing, you have to stretch the muscles, which must be under control. Whichever the adopted position, it is practically impossible to perform the exercise successfully if the back is drooping as is almost always the case with the so-called 'tailor's position' (sitting cross-legged on the ground). If you cannot perform any of the above-mentioned asanas, you may practise sitting on a low chair.

At first, do the exercise incorrectly so that you may have a point of comparison. Empty the lungs as much as possible, contracting the abdominal muscles to expel the air. Now inhale deeply relaxing the abdominal muscles (incorrect) and watch your abdomen protruding like a balloon, which should have been prevented. Next do the exercise correctly. Empty the lungs as before. At the end of the exhalation, the abdomen is firm: keep it this way. Before inhaling, press your left index finger between the navel and the pubis and the right between the navel and the sternum. Press on the abdomen to feel the difference of resistance, still holding your breath with empty lungs. Keeping your fingers in the same place, inhale slowly. Keep the lower part of the abdomen contracted and, during the whole inhalation, let only the area above the navel expand *slightly*. In this manner, the abdominal wall resists the pressure caused by the lowering of the diaphragm which pushes the organs downwards and forward against the abdominal wall. Your fingers will clearly feel the difference of resistance between the two levels of the abdomen. The inhalation requires some muscular effort and that compression is transmitted to the abdominal organs which are massaged vigorously though gently and therefore invigorated.

Effects on thoracic and clavicular breathing
At the end of the exhalation the contracted diaphragm, which opposes the controlled abdomen, has reached its lowest level. You will then notice that the thoracic phase of inhalation starts more easily, more spontaneously and more fully than with relaxed abdominal muscles and distended abdomen. The intercostal muscles, which are a sort of prolongation of the abdominal wall, lift and widen the rib-cage and the thorax expands. The last phase of the respiratory act, the subclavicular phase, starts easily and completes the cycle.

Breath retention with full lungs
Hold your breath, controlling the abdomen and observing the rules for breath retention. It is during breath retention that the increased pressure in abdomen and thorax is most noticeable. The student then feels the need to hold the air within the thorax so that the pressure does not rise above the glottis. This is possible with the help of Jaland-hara Bandha*. Thus the face does not become congested, the pressure remains within the lungs, where it can do no harm because it is evenly distributed over the entire surface of the pulmonary membrane (approximately 140 square metres).

What about ordinary breathing?
The control of the abdomen must not be restricted to pranayama. Normal breathing should be like yoga breathing with abdominal control but in a reduced way. Each time you think of it during the day stiffen the abdomen, especially the area below the navel. When you are driving especially, sit so that you can breathe and control your abdomen. You will thus avoid acquiring a 'spare tyre', for a distended abdomen

---

* See Section 22, p. 133

soon fills up with a roll of fat. This way of breathing will gradually become second nature, or rather a return to nature, since our objective is to regain the abdominal tonus of true natural breathing.

Control but not contraction
The reader might think we are back to 'gymnastic' breathing: 'chest out, abdomen in'. But we are not. There is a world of difference between the two. In gymnastic breathing only thoracic and perhaps clavicular breathing are possible: the diaphragmatic phase, which is essential, is practically omitted.

On the other hand, control is not synonymous with contraction of the abdomen. A contracted abdomen blocks the whole diaphragmatic breathing. A person with high (subclavicular) breathing caused by a taut abdomen, is always anxious and tense, his throat is tight, his solar plexus is contracted; he usually has delicate health, feels the cold, suffers from bad digestion, and is often too thin because of poor food assimilation. He sleeps badly and suffers from frequent headaches. Subclavicular breathing does not ventilate the lungs properly, lowers physical and nervous resistance, and shortens life. Besides, a rigid abdominal wall often corresponds to a constipated intestine (spastic constipation). Asanas can relieve such a person, but only yogic breathing, combined with relaxation, can help him effectively. He must first learn to relax the abdominal muscles at will. When he is less tense and is able to relax the abdominal wall and move the diaphragm, the practice of asanas will bring him maximum benefit. Relaxing the abdomen is the necessary prerequisite for activating the diaphragm, which is blocked in a high position by the contraction of the abdominal wall and the lack of mobility of the ribs. Relaxation of a taut abdomen has spectacular effects: the solar plexus is decongested, breathing is amplified, the spasm in the digestive tract is released, digestion is improved, constipation becomes less stubborn, the feeling of anxiety lessens and disappears, and sleep improves. Such a person must go through the stage of breathing with relaxed abdomen before practising pranayama with abdominal control. All the indications given on this subject in *Yoga Self-Taught*[*] remain valid and concern them especially.

Breathing with distended abdomen

---

[*]   *Yoga Self-Taught*, Chapter 4

Let us see what happens to people who breathe only with distended-abdomens and whose abdominal muscles have become flabby – usually men. This condition has a host of unpleasant consequences.

The organs, no longer supported, practically hang out of the pelvis into the shapeless bag which the abdomen has become. Since the viscera have a larger volume at their disposal, they gorge themselves with an excess of blood and their weight increasingly distends the abdominal cavity. The blocking of the circulation impedes the normal functioning of the organs. The alimentary canal, particularly the colon, becomes obstructed with a useless ballast composed of the accumulated residues of several meals plus pockets of gas. Fat fills the remaining available space. Such people are often constipated but this is due to the lack of tonus in a colon stuffed with waste products which it has no longer the strength to eliminate. One remark in passing: even an ordinary laxative should not be taken indiscriminately. The laxative which acts upon the intestinal mucus membrane to start the contractions of an atonic intestine, when given to a person suffering from spastic constipation, would only aggravate the condition.

Back to breathing with abdominal control. In general persons with distended abdomens do not succeed in contracting the abdominal muscles with the necessary force. They must first strengthen these muscles. As indicated in the Halasana and Sarvangasana techniques, the most efficient yoga exercise consists in pausing at 30 and 60 when raising the legs. Within a few weeks the muscles will regain their tonus and the student will be able to control the abdomen during pranayama.

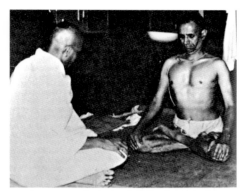

A yoga master in South India (back to the camera) always controls personally the performance of pranayama exercises, even when dealing with the experienced students, as in this case. This is the end of a complete correct yoga inhalation. The lotus is very tight, heels against the abdomen, hands placed on the knees which touch the ground. The pelvis is slightly tilted forward to press the lower part of the abdomen against the heels. The thorax is fully expanded, the abdomen is not distended but controlled. Not a single cubic centimetre of air could be inhaled. Note the position of the retracted chin to facilitate Ujjayi.

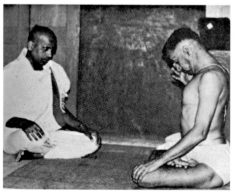

This is the end of a deep inhalation. The student has inhaled through the left nostril and is preparing to hold his breath with full lungs in Jalandhara Bandha. The area above the navel has yielded with elasticity but firmly. The pressure in the abdomen is kept at a high level. The abdomen is not distended but is aligned with the sternum. Study these pictures carefully: they give essential information on the exact evolution of the pranayama exercise. Note particularly the position of the spine.

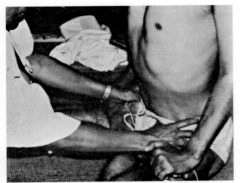

The guru pushes his thumbs into the abdomen (just beside the large straight muscles) to control its tension. This photograph shows a controlled abdomen: it is only the area above the navel that swells up very slightly while the air enters the lungs. We are here in the process of inhalation and about half-way through the diaphragmatic phase.

The aim of pranayama is to increase the absorption and fixation of prana, to accumulate it in specific centres, and then to redistribute this energy throughout the body. In this chapter we shall learn how to 'pranify' our bodies, wholly or in part, at our will. The exercise proposed with this in view is particularly interesting, for it is simple, efficacious and without danger.

Technique
The student assumes a posture suitable for pranayama. Whatever his posture he must make sure before beginning the exercise that his spine is quite straight and upright.

Inhalation (puraka: the absorption phase). During inhalation, which should be slow, uniform and complete, the student should concentrate on the penetration of the air into his nostrils. To facilitate this concentration he may look at the tip of his nose; he will squint a little but must not overdo it, not for fear of strabism but in order not to tire the eye muscles. The eyes will be nearly closed, which will make this fixation of the eyes (a form of tratak) much more agreeable. It is, however, not absolutely essential; it is simply an aid to concentration.

The student should imagine that he is absorbing prana through his nostrils in the form of pure energy. As another aid to concentration he may imagine prana entering his nose as a yellow or blue light. But we must not confuse imagination with illusion. This mental image really helps to fix the prana; thousands of years of yogic experience prove it. Pranayama is a process at once psychic and physical. If the normal fixation of prana were not automatic we should not be alive. From birth our bodies absorb pranic energy from the air without our knowing it, but it is impossible to practise pranayama unconsciously. The yogis' brilliant discovery, perhaps one of the greatest ever made, was that the mind influences the fixation of prana and that we can consciously increase its absorption, fixation and circulation within the body. Pranayama is only possible with the active participation of the mind. This participation consists of concentration and its most effective feature is mental representation, possibly helped by a mantra. From this point of view OM is perfect.

To return to the exercise: while imagining that he is absorbing luminous energy through the nostrils, the yogi is really increasing the amount of prana fixed in his body. I do not know if scientific research has been carried out in this field, but that is unimportant, for we know that by following yogic prescriptions we can secure results. Yogis who use pranayama techniques to stop their hearts beating do not worry whether their methods can be scientifically controlled so long as the results can, thanks, for example, to the electrocardiogram. They have been practising pranayama and benefiting from it for thousands of years without the electrocardiogram, which merely serves for confirmation.

Retention (Khumbaka): the storage phase. At the end of the slow, conscious inhalation, accompanied by the fixation of prana at the level of the nostrils, the student gently holds his breath in his lungs by means of Jalandhara Bandha (see Section 22, p. 133). Meanwhile he concentrates his attention on the pit of his stomach; he may also look at it, for his eyes should not remain fixed on the tip of his nose. During the entire retention period with full lungs the student keeps his mind on this region and, if he can, imagines that he is sending light and energy to it. If he cannot do so, it is not important; the essential thing is to 'interiorise' himself somewhere between the point of the sternum and the navel. After the retention period (the length of which cannot be specified as it depends on the individual and his training) he will first of all perceive pulsations and then reactions of the abdominal wall, especially of the large straight muscles. These reactions will be felt as rhythmic contractions of the muscles, increasing in strength as the retention continues. This khumbaka must be accompanied by Mula Bandha (contraction of the anal and perineal sphincters). These contractions will soon be followed by vibrations in the lower abdomen. During the entire retention period the student concentrates on this region and imagines that he is storing energy there. As soon as retention starts to be uncomfortable, he must pass on to exhalation.

Exhalation (Rechaka): the distribution phase. In this phase the student consciously directs the flow of prana towards the chosen area or lets it diffuse throughout the body. It follows that the exhalation must be prolonged, controlled and complete, which cannot happen if retention has been too long. If exhalation can be controlled so that it is slow and steady then the breath cannot have been retained beyond the student's ability. While the air is slowly escaping through the nostrils (never through the mouth) the student imagines that a current of prana, starting from the region between the sternum and the navel, spreads through his entire body. The rhythmic abdominal con-tractions may continue during exhalation.

If the student for any reason wishes to stimulate a particular limb or organ he may direct the current of prana to that part by imagining that a stream of warmth is moving there. Let us suppose he has sprained an ankle: he may direct the pranic current towards the painful region and after a few minutes he will feel warmth there. The intensity of this experience depends upon the degree of mental concentration, but even with average concentration the sensation of warmth is soon felt.

Repetition. This cycle constitutes one pranayama. It should be repeated several times and the whole exercise should last several minutes. In case of fatigue the exercise may be interrupted for a few normal breaths, but it is essential to keep concentrating on the breathing process even during such interruptions.

Counter-indications.
There are no counter-indications for this exercise since it is just as impossible to overload an organ with prana as it is for one's health to be too good. As an example I quote the case of a woman yoga practitioner who injured both her spine and a kidney in a car crash. She practised this pranic recharge for ten-minute periods several times a day in her hospital bed. To her doctors' astonishment she recovered abnormally fast and suffered no after-effects of the accident.

Psychic effects
This pranayama may be practised without necessarily accepting the pranic theory. I have already alluded to the psychic aspect of pranayama and in this respect the exercise described above is on the dividing line between the physical and the psychic. Its performance will bring great benefits, as the conscious mind is completely absorbed in it and its faculties are reduced, thus benefiting the deepest layers of our consciousness and leading to an awareness of our bodies which is difficult to attain by other means. The body is completely penetrated by consciousness and the physical and mental levels are harmoniously integrated. This pranayama achieves the aim and indeed the very basis

of Hatha Yoga, which is to spiritualise the body. It is the beginning of meditation and its regular practice for only a few minutes a day will lead the student to a state very near to that of deep meditation. Meditation does not mean *doing* something but letting something happen. It is a state and not a series of mental activities. It is no accident that in the Asthanga Yoga of Patanjali pranayama is placed between the asanas and the purely psychic phases of concentration which lead to Samadhi, the supreme integration.

NOTE: Pranic recharging may also be practised while lying down either in the Savasana posture or in bed.

21 | Samavritti Pranayama, The Pranayama Square

This exercise derives its name from the fact that the four phases (inhalation, retention, exhalation, retention) are all of the same duration. It is even more classic and in more general use than the 1:2:4 respiration discussed in most books.

Correct position
Sit in your favourite position for pranayama. As always, the spine must be very straight and the weight of the body must be distributed so that the centre of gravity is in the lower abdomen between the navel and the pubis, when the body will be at ease. In this way the weight will be taken by the hips. It is good to spend some time finding the correct position for the spine so as to ensure a stable and relaxed position which will not provoke secondary muscular contractions. The head, as always, has to be well balanced on top of the spine. Concentrate on the spine as you straighten it, vertebra by vertebra from the sacrum to the top where atlas and axis maintain the skull. Repeat this several times, moving the focus of your concentration alternately upwards and downwards along the spine like a lift. Besides ensuring the comfort of the whole body throughout the exercise, this preliminary concentration creates a state of mental interiorisation essential for the success of all pranayama exercises.

The exercise itself
While normal and habitual respiration only comprises two distinct phases, inhalation (Puraka) and exhalation (Rechaka), yoga adds retention (Khumbaka), which can be practised with the lungs full or with the lungs empty. Khumbaka is essential for pranayama and the pranayama square allows the same amount of time to each of these four phases.

The rhythm
Rhythm is very important for all pranayama exercises. A good rhythm could be obtained simply by counting, say, to six during each phase.

While such a technique is not absolutely wrong, it is much better to establish the rhythm by a series of mental OMS. Concentration on the OM has the advantage of leading to deep mental absorption. You may object that, in order to make a phase last six OMS, it is necessary to count them, which is what we are trying to avoid. This is not so, for it is possible to maintain a definite number of OMS by splitting them into groups without having to count them. Suppose you choose four OMS as your basic rhythm. You then have to repeat two OMS twice. It is easy to listen mentally to OM—OM/OM—OM. For six, listen to OM—OM—OM/OM—OM—OM. It is unnecessary to pause noticeably between the groups of two, three or four OMS. The rhythm establishes itself rapidly and you feel the number of OMS without counting. Quite often you will become aware of your heartbeat during this exercise: you will then be able to regulate your pranayama square by synchronising the OM with your heartbeat. This is the ideal way of controlling your rhythm, but counting OMS is perfectly satisfactory.

The complete exercise
Begin by emptying your lungs completely without counting, then hold your lungs empty while listening to, say, four OMS with the same number of Asvini Mudra contractions (see Section 34). Inhale, at the same time controlling the abdomen, as in the full yoga respiration, and counting four OMS. When the lungs are full, hold your breath and count four OMS, again with Asvini Mudra. Empty your lungs while counting four OMS with the perineum relaxed.

Repeat this cycle as many times as you like without pausing between successive cycles. The number of OMS will depend on the capacity of your lungs. To start with, try the square with four OMS. The exercise is useless with fewer than four and people whose lung capacity is small should first practise complete yoga breathing without retention and without counting. A square of six to eight OMS is the average. You must take time to fill or empty the lungs completely during the active phases. If the timing is correct, you will be able to continue the exercise indefinitely without fatigue. The pranayama square is usually accompanied by Asvini Mudra[*], which is practised during each retention, one contraction accompanying each OM. During inhalation and exhalation the muscles of the perineum are relaxed.

---

[*] See p.186

Here is a diagram of the complete cycle:

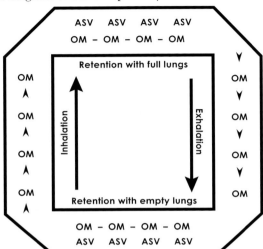

Concentration

Concentration is essential for maximum effectiveness. The mind has to be strictly concentrated on pranayama, avoiding all distractions. At the beginning distractions are normal, but we must continually bring the mind back to the exercise without being discouraged. After a little while the mind will become completely absorbed and this is one of the objects of this pranayama. It is, in fact, an ideal preparation for meditation. How must we concentrate, and where should we direct the attention?

During inhalation concentrate on the OMS and on the air streaming into the nasal cavities; the air should be directed as high as possible. *During retention with full lungs* concentrate on the OMS and on the contractions of Asvini Mudra and, if possible, on your heartbeats too, if this can be done without loss of concentration on Asvini Mudra. *During exhalation* concentrate on the movement of the warm air passing through the nostrils and on the OMS. *During retention with empty lungs* concentrate on the OMS and on Asvini Mudra (as for retention with full lungs).

Variation

Instead of concentrating on the movement of air through the nostrils the exercise may be practised in Ujjayi, concentrating on the sound of the air in the throat caused by the slight contraction of the glottis.

Duration of the exercise
The pranayama square may be practised as long as it is agreeable and as long as the student wishes and is able to concentrate. If t h e pranayama tires or bores him, he must stop and begin again later. It may be practised at any time except immediately after a meal.

As the exercise loses much of its value when the mind no longer concentrates, it is necessary to guard against its becoming mechanical or automatic. The mind has to be as clear as possible, even during the phase of absorption. Drowsiness is a 'technical hitch' to be avoided, since it prevents the student from crossing a certain threshold impossible to describe but very easily recognised when it is reached. Once there the mind is in a special state; the student remains perfectly conscious of all the phases of the exercise, concentrated and absorbed, but he no longer hears any outside sound or he hears sounds so weakly that they no longer disturb his concentration. The mechanism of the inner verbalism which makes us talk to ourselves mentally when awake is disconnected, and our consciousness is no longer disturbed by extraneous thought.

We have only to advance one step further to enter into the state of meditation where we acquire the ability to observe our own minds and bodies as if from a distance. The student is no longer *in* his mind but *behind* it and he no longer identifies with himself. The perception of the deep Self, of the Spectator who transcends time, space and tht limits of the physical body, may occur at this level.

Advantages of the pranayama square
Right from the start, even before you are able to carry it out perfectly you will realise how complete and efficient this exercise is. It includes rhythm, a Mudra, mental concentration, the OM, breath retention and control of the vital processes. It is without danger if the rule of absolute comfort during retention is respected. If you can continue the exercise indefinitely you are assured of never unwittingly outstripping your respiratory capacity. It trains the lungs for prolonged retentions by gentle progression and thus without danger. You must not forget that rhythm and concentration are infinitely more important than retention time expressed in seconds. With a little practice you will discover your own

rhythm most suited to the deepest concentration, the greatest ease which strengthens rather than tires.

From the pranic viewpoint this is an incomparable exercise. It automatically redistributes the prana in the dense as well as in the subtle body. Only Muladhara Chakra appears to be stimulated by Asvini Mudra. Nevertheless, all the subtle centres of pranic and psychic energy are uniformly recharged, which is of great importance for our psycho-physical balance.

Some authors condemn any concentration on the so-called lower centres situated below the heart, especially those situated near the base of the spine. They may not be completely wrong, for it is possible that very prolonged and strong concentration on these regions may produce unfortunate results if the student has no guru. These authors fear a sudden 'awakening' of 'Kundalini', the mysterious one. But Kundalini is not so easily awakened. Kundalini is a latent energy present in every living being just as there is an enormous intra-atomic energy in even the most ordinary pebble on your garden path. This is a scientific fact. Another fact, just as scientific, is that it is theoretically possible to liberate this energy. Disintegrating through the sudden liberation of these energies, the pebble could reduce your house to a ruin. Theoretically this is a real danger, but in practice it does not exist. Parents can let their children play with the pebbles in the garden without fear of an atomic explosion. Yogis whom I have questioned on this subject agreed that such concentration as we have described is without danger; very few had reservations and they could not specify the exact dangers which a Westerner would encounter.

From my own personal experience and those of my numerous pupils I can confirm that I have never felt anything other than the flowering of a new healthy and balanced dynamism and a true spirituality. You should practise this exercise regularly every day, preferably after a session of asanas, because the asanas are the ideal preparation for pranayama. In the Ashtanga Yoga of Patanjali, pranayama immediately follows the asanas. This does not mean that one must have mastered all the asanas before practising any pranayama exercise but rather that in the series of exercises pranayama logically follows the asanas. These prepare the body for an increased pranic circulation and allow a better revitalisation of the whole human being, including the psyche. You can practise the Pranayama square without fear!

'Bandha', like so many words of the yogic vocabulary, cannot be translated exactly into Western languages. It means to tie, to control, to block, to hold, to join and to contract, all at the same time. In yoga practice, and particularly in pranayama, Bandha refers to various muscular contractions intended to influence the circulation of the blood, the nervous system and the endocrine glands. Most Bandhas are concerned with the control of one particular orifice of the body.

From the yogic point of view, the purpose of the Bandhas is to awaken and control the subtle pranic energy present in our bodies. We have already studied Uddiyana Bandha (not to be confused with Uddiyana) in detail. Jalandhara Bandha is probably the most important Bandha associated with pranayama as it necessarily accompanies all prolonged breath retentions (Kumbhaka with full lungs).

Etymology
'Jala' means net, network, trellis: 'The chin must be pressed against the chest so as to close the network of arteries in the neck; this is what is referred to as the Contraction of the Network* which is difficult even for the gods.' This is quoted from Shiva Samhita IV, 60-62, by Alain Danielou, who adds: 'The chin is pressed against the triangular hollow formed at the junction of the collar bones and this causes pressure on the Centre of Extreme Purity (Vishudda Chakra) situated in the neck. Properly done, this contraction blocks the respiratory apparatus and, when the breath is held (Kumbhaka), it prevents the air causing pressure above the glottis.' Other authors say Jala means 'nerves which pass through the neck towards the brain'.

'Dhara' means pulling upwards.

Technique
Hatha-Yoga Pradipika describes the technique summarily in verses III, 70–71: 'Having contracted the throat, the student will press his chin firmly on the chest. This Bandha, which prevents premature ageing and death, is called Jalandhara because it compresses the arteries which lead to the brain and stops the nectar from flowing downwards.'

---

* The network mentioned here is a network of nadis.

Although this text is familiar, it is not generally known that Jalandhara is mentioned in the Upanishads (Yoga-Chudamany- Upanishad, Sloka 51): 'Thanks to Jalandhara Bandha, which contracts the cavity of the throat, the nectar which descends from the Lotus of the Thousand Petals [the brain] is not consumed by the digestive fire so that it can control the vital forces and awaken Kundalini.' According to these descriptions it would be sufficient to contract the throat muscles and to put the chin against the chest in order to accomplish Jalandhara, but in fact it is not quite so simple. We must remember that the classic treatises of Hatha Yoga were written not as detailed technical manuals but as résumés.

Jalandhara may be practised at any stage of the respiratory act, but we shall describe it only as practised with full lungs. Inhale, hold your breath and swallow your saliva. At the completion of the act of swallowing, contract the throat muscles, block them and place the chin in the fork of the sternum (the concave notch in the upper part of the sternum between the collar bones). It is essential to place the chin correctly at this precise spot in order to achieve one of the main objectives of Jalandhara, the stretching of the cervical vertebrae, and to ensure the ideal compression of the neck. The three key points are: 1 compression of the throat; 2 contraction of the neck muscles; 3 stretching of the cervical vertebrae. The neck muscles remain contracted during the whole of Jalandhara Bandha. It will be found impossible to breathe in or out since Jalandhara Bandha really seals the breath in the chest. This impossibility is moreover a test of the correctness of Jalandhara Bandha.

In some cases Jalandhara Bandha is held during inhalation or exhalation. It is then necessary to relax it a little and to free the glottis so as to leave a passage for the air. This can produce the characteristic sound of Ujjayi (see p. 164).

When should we use Jalandhara Bandha?
As we have said, Jalandhara may accompany all phases of pranayama but *it must always accompany any prolonged breath retention*. Jalandhara practised in combination with Mula Bandha and Uddiyana constitutes 'Bandha Traya', the Triple Bandha.

Why Jalandhara?
From the yogic point of view, Jalandhara Bandha modifies the pranic

current in sixteen vital centres but it is unnecessary to go into more detail here. Prana is directed towards the centres situated near the base of the spine. We shall go into this when we study the Chakras. For the moment the following physiological explanations will suffice to justify the practice of Jalandhara, the effects of which are:

1   *It seals off the breath in the chest.* During breath retention with full lungs we could keep the inhaled air inside by pinching the nose while keeping the head straight, without blocking the glottis. Try this and see what happens (there is no danger if you do this occasionally as an experiment), and let the air pressure exert itself right up to the nostrils. You will feel a particular sensation in the ears, which will not surprise you because nose, ears and throat are linked. In the practice of pranayama it is absolutely essential to avoid the development of pressure beyond the glottis, especially in the Eustachian tubes. This is absolutely forbidden. It is possible to block the breath, without bending the head, by contracting the throat and the glottis. This is sufficient for short retentions. For long retentions Jalandhara, a safety lock, seals the breath in the chest.

2   *It acts on the heart.* During breath retention the heart must not beat too quickly. On the contrary, the beating must slow down to a strong, calm and regular rhythm.

In order to understand how Jalandhara Bandha steadies the heart's activity, we must study the neck, a strategic region containing an impressive number of arteries, veins and nerve centres, not forgetting the thyroid gland, which we shall consider later. It would need several chapters to deal fully with this subject, so we shall deal only with the essentials.

Everybody knows that the carotid artery passes through the neck and that it is the most important blood vessel supplying the brain. In fact there are three carotid arteries on each side of the neck. These are branches of the original carotid. In the neck the main artery bifurcates and thus forms the carotid sinus which has very thin walls and is thus extremely sensitive to any pressure. Nerves start from the carotid sinuses – one on each side of the neck – and the yogis know that by pressing on this spot the activity of the brain, and with it the state of consciousness, can be considerably modified. The Siva Samhita (V,55) describes a very dangerous practice which may be carried out only under the direct personal supervision of a guru. We quote this text in order to show that the yogis of ancient India had a very precise knowledge of the psycho-physiological repercussions of Jalandhara Bandha: 'The yogi must compress the two carotid nerves (on either side of the neck). Then the pure Brahman appears and the adept knows happiness.'

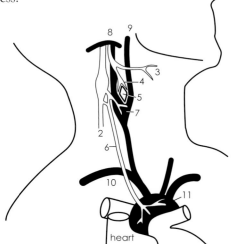

1. plexiform ganglion
2. vagus or nerve
3. glossopharyngeal nerve
4. carotid sinus nerve
5. intercarotid plexus
6. cardiocervical ramifications
7. carotid sinus
8. internal carotid artery
9. external carotid artery
10. subclavian artery
11. aorta

Physiology teaches us that the carotid sinus nerves are very sensitive transmitters of any change of pressure in this region, and that any increase of pressure produces, as a reflex action, a reduction of arterial pressure and a slowing down of the heartbeats. Now the effect of prolonged breath retention is to increase the arterial pressure and to produce an acceleration of the heartbeat that might cause palpitations. Jalandhara Bandha thus serves to protect the heart and the vascular system from any ill effects of prolonged breath retention.

This is the physiological explanation of Jalandhara. The yogis found that pressure on the carotid sinus nerve, in addition to influencing blood pressure and heartbeat, creates a state of oblivion which is neither torpor nor fainting but rather a state of hypnotic trance. 'When controlled by experts this trance "interiorises" human awareness and extrasensory perception becomes possible. Spiritual worlds reveal their secrets and individual awareness becomes more and more refined until this perception reaches a point where individual awareness disappears and the individual merges with the infinite."[*] The mechanical compression which the yogis practise with their fingers must be so slight as to touch only the nerve; compression of the artery must be avoided as it would stop the supply of blood to the brain which, if prolonged, could cause irreparable damage. As practised by the yogis, the compression of the nerve hardly affects the irrigation of the brain and can therefore cause no damage.

In Jalandhara Bandha, the contraction of the neck muscles acts gently on the nerves and the phenomena mentioned above occur at only a very low level. Jalandhara allows us to feel the circulation of prana and calms the mind. The description of the various states of consciousness given above should neither frighten nor attract you. In practice they occur only after such long training that they are inaccessible to most Westerners through lack of available training.

3 *It stretches the cervical region of the spine.* When the chin is correctly placed in the fork of the sternum, the student notices a stretching of the nape of the neck – of the cervical vertebrae – which extends even to the back muscles. If the rest of the spine is in the correct position, this stretching of the nape of the neck pulls on the spinal cord and thereby stimulates all the rachidian nervous centres. Thanks to Jalandhara the stretching of the cervical vertebrae frees the important cranial nerves and acts on the cephalo-rachidian bulb. This bulb contains the respiratory and cardiac centres which control the vasomotor nerves and certain essential metabolisms. It is the vital centre where a pinprick kills! It is also the starting-point of the parasympathetic nerve. Jalandhara thus acts through the stretched position of the neck on the respiratory centre which is strongly excited during breath retention. Without considering further anatomical details, which would only interest specialists, the student will grasp the importance of Jalandhara and realise the deep repercussions which this Bandha causes in all these areas. He can have confidence in the yogis and accompany any breath retention by Jalandhara Bandha.

4 *It compresses the thyroid.* The compression of the neck by the chin has an important affect on the thyroid gland. People known to suffer from an overactive thyroid (they will be under treatment as a disorder

---

[*]   Yoga Mimansa IV, 316

of the thyroid does not pass unnoticed) must not practise Jalandhara or even pranayama. They may, however, practise complete yogic breathing and this is even desirable.

Jalandhara Bandha and Sarvangasana with Halasana

The practice of the asanas must necessarily precede pranayama. Jalandhara Bandha can only be carried out correctly and without fatigue if the student practises Sarvangasana (the shoulder stand) and Halasana (the plough) regularly. These two postures automatically lead to the Jalandhara position and the stretching of the neck. Students who practise pranayama must devote more time to these two postures and carry them out in a more advanced manner, that is by placing their hands as near the shoulder-blades as possible and pulling the elbows towards each other in order to bring the cervical vertebrae perpendicular to the rest of the spine.

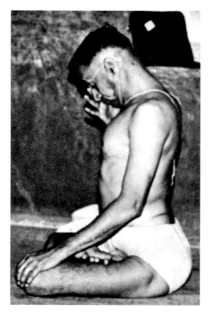

This adept of Ashtanga Yoga Nilayam of Mysore is demonstrating Jalandhara Bandha, which enhances the spine's own curvature so as to pull on the spinal cord. The correct position of the pelvis is obtained in the lotus position with both knees touching the floor. The neck muscles are strongly contracted during Jalandhara. The chin is placed in the fork of the sternum and not on the sternum itself.

23 | The Nadis

I am reminded at this point of those examinations when at school I sat facing a blank sheet of paper, chin in hand and my eyes roaming over the ceiling as I waited in vain for inspiration. But right now it is not lack of inspiration which prevents me from starting but the com-plex-ity of a subject as vast as the nadis, comprising notions so very different from those of the West. Paradoxically, fifteen years ago I should not have hesitated so long before writing this section. In fact, basing my statements on the work of Dr Vasant G. Rele, such as his book *The Mysterious Kundalini*, in which he tries to match classical physiology and anatomy with those of the yogic treatises, I should probably have written that the nadis of the yogis can be likened to the nerves and the chakras to the various plexi of our bodies, which would have been both true and false at the same time.

Starting from the assumption that two distinct physiologies can-not exist together, I then thought it possible to make the yogic ideas of nadis and chakras correspond with our present-day knowledge of anatomy and physiology, but today I am much less sure of this. I am in-clined to think that a scientific physiology of the Western type, based on observation and objective measurement, of which no one can deny the rigour, can coexist with a different though parallel anatomy and physiology. Lacking any other valid hypothesis, it seemed clear to me that when the classic Sanskrit texts talked of 72,000 nadis circulat-ing energy throughout the body they meant the nerves and that the energy they convey are the nerve impulses. Continuing my interest in the matter I studied other ancient texts, where I found categorical statements which excluded the hypothesis that the nadis were the nerves.

The doubts that entered my mind did not stop me from practising pranayama according to yogic techniques nor from feeling the effects I had expected. I wondered whether to avoid the question and omit the problem of the nadis and chakras, since in any case the exercises would lose nothing of their value or effectiveness. However, I do not believe I have the right to do so, for the subject is of capital importance for an understanding of the way pranayama acts.

Let us first see how I ceased identifying the nadis with the nerves. Dr M. V. Apte of the Institute of Lonavla writes in a noteworthy study,

Nadis in Yoga:

'The nadis provide a fertile theme for yogic literature. It is also disconcerting. Some texts seem to show that nadis are nerves, while others clearly indicate that this is not so. There are discrepancies between the treatises and, sometimes even in the same work, starting from the hypothesis that the nadis are the nerves, we find passages which contradict this.'

Elsewhere Dr Apte is even more categorical: 'Any attempt to give an anatomical meaning to this [the nadis and the chakras] is bound to fail.' This is clear.

Another writer, whom I consider to be an authority, the Lama Anagarika Govinda, writes in his remarkable work, *Les Fondements de la mystique tibétaine*: 'The nadis cannot be identified with the nerves… The translations have caused misunderstandings. The nadis are neither veins nor arteries nor nerves.' So what are they? If the treatises cannot agree, perhaps it would be better to turn the page and deal with other subjects. Perhaps, in fact, it is a discussion of only academic significance. But I am, on the contrary, convinced of its immense importance, and I agree with the Lama Govinda that 'All attempts show that yoga cannot be measured by the standards of anatomy, of physiology based on dissection, or of experimental psychology.'

Yogic anatomy is essentially dynamic in that it describes dynamic processes which are both physiological and psychological rather than anatomical structures. It is based on introspection rather than on exterior observation of structures. With such a dynamic conception of the physiology of the nadis, the contradictions disappear. If, as we have already shown, prana is electrical energy – negative ions – not excluding other forms such as the micromagnetic fields in the human body, and if we consider the pranic body as the sum total of all these energies, the nadis are all the conductors of this energy and, whatever they may be, these conductors can be very varied.

The prana in the air can act directly on the nerve endings of the nose and pass with the air into the lungs where it is absorbed by the blood. It can circulate with the blood in the arteries, capillaries and veins and, carried by the blood to the brain, it can become the motor of activities of the neurons and circulate as nervous energy along the nerves. With this dynamic conception of prana and the nadis it is no longer necessary to limit the circulation of prana to a particular type of conductor such as nerves, veins or arteries. The treatises no longer contradict one another and their statements become complementary. The nerves are certainly conductors of prana but they are not the only ones.

Some Western scientists have known intuitively of this bioenergy which yoga calls 'prana' and have tried to measure it experimentally. They have partially succeeded, in particular Wilhelm Reich, a controversial figure not so much because of his theories as because of his planned commercial exploitation of these theories. He writes: 'Transmission of bio-energy cannot be limited to the nervous system alone. We must admit that this energy follows all the membranes and all the fluids of the body.'

In an appendix to Hime's translation of *The Thirteen Upanishads*, Dr George G. D. Hass writes:

'It is clear that when using the term "nadi" the authors of the Upanishads had in mind the same vessels that were later described in such detail in the writings on yoga and other subjects. These treatises consider the nadis as channels for the circulation of vital energies, specialised in different ways in the etheric or spiritual vehicle which exists in counterpart to the dense body, in that composite structure, the human body.'

There must also be a relationship between the nadis of yoga and the meridians of acupuncture.

Some authors do not agree with these texts. They think, and I agree with them, that the nadis are a physical part of the human body and therefore visible, tangible and material. I cannot see any contradiction here. The pranic body must not be considered as a 'spirit' or some immaterial phantom. It is material, just as electricity is material, although invisible, except in its manifestations and its conductors, the electric cables and wires.

The ancient Upanishads, especially Chandogya and Brihadara-ranyaka, say of the nadis: 'The subtle body is a group of seventeen constituents which are in these nadis.' We can understand this text if we distinguish between the energy and its carriers. The energy, prana, is part of the subtle body, while the carriers are part of the dense body which can be dissected with a scalpel.

Western anatomy is objective. It describes the visible and tangible structures: it dissects, isolates and classifies. Yogic anatomy is not based on the dissection of dead bodies. It is subjective and is centred on interior observation of processes taking place in the living and conscious human body.

The yogis, thanks to an extremely refined mental concentration which they direct towards the physiological processes of their own organisms, obscure the entrance of prana and are able to follow its passage within themselves. They perceive directly how it is transformed, how it circulates and how it accumulates. This energy may use a series of real and objective physiological and anatomical carriers which may be very different from one another. The yogis make no distinction between the different carriers. To return to the example of electrical energy in a house: it not only travels along wires; it can be converted to luminous energy in a lamp bulb. It can also return through an earth wire, circulate along the water pipes and vanish into the earth, absorbed by its negative mass. If we can visualise this energy and follow it, we do so without considering the carriers used.

In the Upanishads mentioned above (Brihadaranyaka, IV, 3 -20) it says: 'The human being possesses these nadis. They are as fine as a hair split into 1,000 and they are filled with white, blue, yellow, red or green liquid.'

Summary
We can therefore argue that the nadis: a) are distributed throughout the physical body; b) do not extend outside the body (thus they are anatomic and material); c) are distinct from the pranic body although the pranic body remains and functions within them.

Shiva Samhita (II, 18) gives a description of the nadis which compares them to the fibres of the lotus (which impregnate the whole plant) and maintains that they descend the length of the spine which supports them. He also mentions their roots. Consequently we may think of them as anatomical structures and we can agree that they also represent nerves. The etymology of the word 'nadi' must not be forgotten, for the word means canal, conduit or tube. 'In Gheranda Samhita, the nadis are the channels which conduct the invigorating energy of the air to the places where it is used in vital processes, whatever their anatomical situation. We know a great number of vital processes which involve arteries, veins and nerves at the same time but it is impossible to identify the nadis with any one of these structures.'*

As the aim of pranayama is the conscious and voluntary control of the subtle energies which circulate within the human body, it is important to know where these energies circulate and especially what are their principal channels of circulation.

---

* Kuvalayananda, Swami & Shukla: *Gorakshasatakam*, *Kayvalyadhama Samiti*, Lonavla. 1958.

Yogic physiology, based on introspective – and thus subjective – observation of processes taking place within the living body, is far from simple. Western science mistrusts subjective data, and often with good reason, but in the case of pranayama this method was the only one available to the yogis for studying the subtle currents of prana within their own bodies. For example, there are two ways of discovering the sciatic nerve. The Western method consists of dissecting a dead body and following the path of the nerve for its whole length. This method is objective and indisputable. The other method is used – unwillingly – by the victims of sciatica; they 'feel' the path of the nerve along the leg right down to the big toe because the nerve is irritated. The yogis, developing their powers of internal perception, have noticed the circulation of energy within their bodies along the nadis. Their subtle physiology is based on this internal observation, and in this way they have been able to portray the nadis graphically.

Let us look at two drawings of the nadis and the chakras. The first is reassuringly simple. It is the frontispiece of that great work by Arthur Avalon, *The Serpent Power*, and it will have been seen by readers of many different works on pranayama.

The other drawing, entitled 'Pranayama', is an ancient parchment showing the main nadis and the positions of those vital points, the chakras. It gives a good idea of the complexity of the subject and of the development of the yogis' knowledge of the circulation of subtle energies within the body. This drawing must not be taken as a strict anatomical representation of the nadis as we know that they are situated *within* the body. The author has drawn the nadis outside the body for reasons of clarity. Thus, what is portrayed is not the exact paths but the correspondence between the lines of force, their beginnings and their distribution centres (chakras). And we must remember that the nadis are very numerous. Apart from the figure of 72,000 already mentioned, some treatises say there are over 350,000 (Shiva Samhita). No one has counted them and these figures must not be taken literally any more than the number of asanas, which is supposed to be 84,000 (or 8,400,000?). In a very important text (Gorakshasataka of the Nath sect) the guru Goraknath says: 'There are as many asanas as there are living creatures. Only Mahesvara [the Supreme Being] knows all their varieties. Of the 84 lakhs [one lakh = 100,000] only 84 are useful to man.' Probably the masters of that time taught 84 main asanas but, to emphasise that their choice was not restrictive, they maintained that there were many more, in fact 100,000 times more! It is just the same with the nadis.

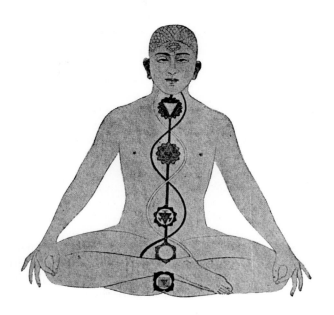

In this drawing the nadis Ida and Pingala intertwine and coil around Sushumna like the two serpents round Aesculapius' staff. This drawing has been reproduced many times in yogic literature. Anagarika Govinda, in the work quoted in Section 23, insists twice on the fact that in Tibetan tradition there is never any question of a spiral path of Ida and Pingala.

Without going too deeply into the subject of nadis, we must try to clarify it a little, especially as there are many contradictions in the classic texts. These contradictions need not worry us unduly as they are often due to inadequate translation of the original texts. Sanskrit experts who make these translations are not necessarily yoga experts so they may not quite realise what the author had in mind. In their defence it must be said that these texts are often purposely made obscure and incomprehensible to the non-initiated. It is therefore not surprising that disagreements exist.

However, if we keep to essentials – and that suffices for our purpose – the writings agree. Let us go back to Gorakshasataka. Verses 17-23 concern the nadis:

17   'Among the thousands of nadis which serve as carriers of prana, seventy-two are said to be important. Of these, ten are particularly noteworthy:

18   'Ida and Pingala and the third one, Sushumna, the others being Ghandari, Hastijihva, Pusha and Yashasvini.

19   'Alambusha, Kuhu and Shankini, the tenth. The yogis should always know this network of nadis.

20   'Ida is situated on the left, Pingala on the right and Sushumna in the middle. Ghandari ends at the left eye.

21   'Hastijihva ends at the right eye. Pusha ends at the right ear. Yashasvini reaches the left ear and Alambusha ends in the mouth.

22   'Kuhu is situated above the penis, Shankini in the Muladhara [anus]. The ten nadis and their ends are thus situated and each one is a path of prana.

23   'The nadis Ida, Pingala and Sushumna carry prana continuously. They are described as being ruled by their divinities which are the Moon, the Sun and Fire.'

The Westerner must remember the last three especially and know that the seven others are linked to the body orifices and the sense organs: the eyes, the nostrils, the ears, the mouth, the anus and the genital orifice. These are the main nadis. The tenth, Sushumna, which runs through the body from the anus to the top of the head, is the most important. The three essential nadis are Ida and Pingala, which start from the nostrils, and Sushumna. The texts agree that Ida is on the left (left nostril) and Pingala on the right (right nostril). They descend along the spine to reach the common starting-point of all the nadis, Kandha 'which is egg-shaped and is situated between the penis and the navel' (sacrum?). Ida links the left testicle (or left ovary) to the left nostril by a pranic circuit running along the spinal column on the left. Ida is lunar and is also called Chandra Nadi (Chandra = moon: *Ha*). Pingala, its opposite number on the right, is the sun nadi (*Tha* = Surya Nadi). This takes us back to the idea of polarity. Most writers agree that Sushumna is situated in Merudanda, which is the spine. We shall limit our present discussion to Ida and Pingala and we shall study Sushumna separately as it is of the greatest importance from the point of view of pranayama. The fact that Ida and Pingala begin in the nostrils shows their special role in pranayama as they control the main openings which allow prana to enter the human body.

In terms of Western anatomy and physiology one could identify Ida and Pingala with the nerves that run from the nostrils to the brain and then, after a complicated path, follow the two chains of sympathetic ganglions right down the spinal column.

Sushumna can perhaps be identified with the spinal cord. There is one doubt in this reasoning, as Sushumna starts at the anus which the spinal cord does not reach, but if we consider that the nerves which control the anal sphincter are in contact with the spine through the pelvic parasympathetic nerve, we must admit that a link exists between the anus and the brain via the spinal cord. Whether these nadis do in fact coincide with the sympathetic nervous system and the spinal cord is of relatively little importance for the practice of pranayama, as the techniques 'work' the way they have been described. It is only on an academic level that we are concerned with the possible correspondence with anatomical structures. Future research may suggest other anatomical routes for Ida, Pingala and Sushumna, but that will not change the practice of pranayama in the least.

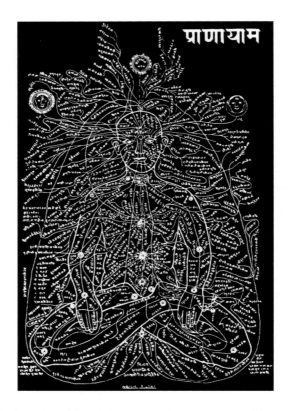

On this ancient parchment the chakras are much more numerous. Ida and Pingala do
not cross Sushumna. They follow a path parallel to the spine

2 5 | K a p a l a b h a t i

Although the Shastras* classify Kapalabhati as belonging to the Shat Kriyas (purification procedures) this exercise is in practice an integral part of pranayama. It is one of the great classics which every student must know and practise.

Etymology
The name can be split into Kapalat**, which means skull, and Bhati, a Sanskrit root meaning to make shiny, to clean. Kapalabhati literally means 'cleaning the skull'. In this case skull means the nostrils, the ears and the other air ducts inside the head.

Technique
Before describing the technique in detail, I must point out that several variations exist, of which three are described in Gheranda Samhita. The number of variations in existence shows the importance of the exercise. I shall describe the two variations which are most commonly practised. The description of the basic exercise given here is the one I studied at the Kuvalyadhama of Lonavla.

Résumé of the exercise and preliminary remarks. In contrast with normal respiration where inhalation is active and exhalation passive, in Kapalabhati exhalation is active, while inhalation is passive. Moreover, in other pranayama exercises exhalation is slower than inhalation (generally twice as long). In Kapalabhati this is inverted. Kapalabhati consists of the forced expulsion of air in short bursts each of which is followed by a passive inhalation.

Position. When carried out in moderation, the exercise may be practised in any position recommended for pranayama, i.e. siddhasana, vajrasana or the lotus. When practised in its more advanced forms and particularly when it aims at attaining certain spiritual objectives, the lotus position is essential. The hands should be in the Jnana Mudra

---

* Classic yoga writings such as the Hatha Yoga Pradipika and the Gheranda Sarnhita.

** This is pronounced *kapala* with the accent on the second syllable and a silent a at the end. Note the resemblance to the Latin *caput* = head.

(see Section 29). Exceptionally the exercise may be practised standing up. The spine must be straight and the head well balanced.

The thorax. Kapalabhati is a purely diaphragmatic or abdominal pranayama. Nevertheless the thorax plays an important part, precisely that of staying completely immobile. Before starting Kapalabhati throw out your chest and hold it in the inhalation position with ribs distended. It must stay as immobile as possible during the whole exercise; this is essential for success. If you watch the thorax during the exercise, you will see that, although it is blocked, the lower ribs move. This movement, which is inevitable and passive, is due to the pull of the abdominal muscles which are linked ro the ribs. Any voluntary and active movement of the thorax must be avoided.

The abdomen. The abdomen is the motor of the exercise. You must ignore the indications given in Section 19 for the control of the abdomen during breathing. The control required for Kapalabhati is totally different. Settle in your favourite position with a straight spine and your chest blocked when full of air and concentrate on what is happening in your abdomen. The centre of gravity of your body must be in the lower abdomen below the navel. Relax the abdomen so that it protrudes. Next, contract the muscles of the abdomen, especially the large straight ones, sharply. This contraction will cause a violent expulsion of air. Relax the abdomen immediately but slowly; the abdomen will again protrude slightly as air enters the lungs passively and silently.

Kapalabhati consists of a rapid succession of such sharp expulsions of air followed by passive inhalation. During this passive inhalation, take care to control the relaxation of the abdomen gradually so that the air enters relatively slowly. The duration of the expulsion is about two-tenths of a second, whereas inhalation varies between eight-tenths and three-tenths according to the rhythm of execution (see below).

How can we judge whether the expulsion of air is sufficiently forceful and brief? Look at your nostrils, which must be relaxed. At the moment of expulsion they open visibly and at once. They do not move during inhalation. The abdomen moves swiftly during contraction so as to compress the lower abdomen in the direction of the sacrum. It is mainly the part below the navel that acts. You should not try to pull the belt in so as to get rid of more air at each expulsion, as it is not the quantity of expelled air that is important, but the force with which it is expelled. The amount is hardly more than that exhaled during normal respiration. You can ensure such force by imagining that you are giving a staggering blow with the muscular abdominal belt at the part below the navel. At first you may make the mistake of pushing the abdomen back as far as possible or of retracting it.

Another way of checking whether the expulsion of air is correct involves the use of a mirror. Stand in front of it and watch what happens at the base of the neck and in the hollows below the collar-bones (the 'salt cellars'). If the expulsion is sufficiently forceful, you will see a lifting of the salt cellars and a brief swelling at the base of the neck, because the lungs are pushed upwards by the diaphragm which is itself pushed upwards. Start a new and strong exhalation followed by a passive inhalation with progressive relaxation of the abdomen. Kapalabhati consists of a short or long series of such expulsions.

Rhythm. The quality of the exercise depends on the force of exhalation; the number of these per minute is of secondary consideration. Increase the speed gradually, first to sixty exhalations a minute, and then to a maximum of 120 per minute. This is the maximum tolerated at Lonavla although I have seen the exercise practised faster. The objection at Lonavla, with which I agree, is that by increasing the speed beyond 120 per minute, some of the force of the exercise is lost.

Error. Many people find that the length of the exhalation tends to equal that of the following inhalation. This (with the retention of the abdomen) is the most common error. This error reduces the force of the exercise and thereby its usefulness. The inhalation should last at least three times as long as the expulsion.

Control of the glottis. There are two ways of controlling the direction of the expelled air, one by directing it into the nostrils; the noise is almost the same as when you blow your nose without a handkerchief, and it is advisable to hold an open handkerchief below the nose. When practised in this way the exercise justifies its name 'cleansing the skull'. It should be continued until no mucus comes out of the nostrils. If the exercise is continued longer, as is recommended for the purposes of pranayama, the expulsion must be controlled and a brake applied at the glottis. The glottis should not be contracted as strongly as in Ujjayi but much more gently. The exhalation of air then makes a slight noise in the throat instead of in the nostrils. Inhalation is silent. By trying gently you will find the right technique.

Progressive training. The other basic element of Kapalabhati is the number of exhalations per group. Here, too, you must not try to run before you can walk. Kapalabhati is a vigorous exercise; the lungs have to get used to it slowly. During the first week you should carry out groups of ten exhalations (each followed by slowed-down inhalation). After the first group, rest for thirty seconds while breathing slowly and easily. Carry out three groups of ten in this way. Add another ten exhalations to the group each week until you finally reach groups of 120, lasting one minute, each group being followed by a rest period of one minute. Three groups of 120 exhalations constitute a good measure. In India, the yogis increase this to several hundred.

If we compare Kapalabhati with normal respiration which takes place at the rate of twenty per minute we see that the speed is increased sixfold. Kapalabhati is an exercise in abdominal breathing but on a superficial level.

Applications
Kapalabhati should be practised at the beginning of each session of pranayama, and even at the beginning of a session of asanas, to get rid of all the air remaining in the lungs and to ensure a good oxygenation of the blood (see 'Effects', p. 154).

Concentration
At the beginning concentrate on the correct execution of the exercise: the force of expulsion, the slowing down of inhalation, the speed of performance, keeping the chest immobile and expanded, and relaxation of the face (do not grimace!). Later concentrate on the part of the abdomen below the navel and on the point of impact of the muscular contraction at the moment of exhalation. Continue to concentrate on this part of the body during the rest periods.

Bandhas
Breaths follow one another without interruption. As there are no retentions, do not practise Jalandhara Bandha. If you practise the exercise intensively (for several minutes running), Mula Bandha will begin

automatically, even without conscious effort on your part. This means that you are carrying the exercise out correctly, but do not perform the Bandha voluntarily.

Counter-indications

Kapalabhati is subject to the same restrictions as all pranayama exercises. Anyone suffering from a lung condition must not practise it. Those who suffer from heart trouble may practise Kapalabhati, but only after a long preparatory period of respiration with control of the abdominal muscles. Strictly speaking, emphysema is no counter-indication, as any part that has been permanently affected cannot be made worse by Kapalabhati. However, emphysema indicates that the lungs are very fragile and that great prudence is necessary.

Recapitulation

Position. Siddhasana, vajrasana or the lotus (the lotus is indispensable for intensive practice). Spine straight, head well balanced. Chest expanded, ribs distended in the inhalation position during the whole exercise.

The exercise. The swift vigorous contraction of the abdominal muscles expels the air. Controlled relaxation of the abdominal muscles causes passive inhalation. These are the only muscles active during Kapalabhati. Relaxation of the face, particularly of the nostrils. Inhalation takes three times as long as expulsion of the air. Practice must be divided into groups, progressive both in number and in speed, to reach three groups of 120 expulsions per minute separated by rest periods.

Errors: letting the chest take part in the exercise; lifting the shoulders; equalising the duration of expulsion and inhalation; pulling in the abdomen; not keeping the spine completely straight and immobile; practising absent-mindedly; sacrificing the force of expulsion to speed.

Variations with alternate respiration

In Kapalabhati, as described above, the nostrils stay open. Kapalabhati may also be practised with alternate respiration, which brings all its advantages. There are two versions of Kapalabhati with alternate respiration:

Variation I . Practise Kapalabhati as described above but block the left nostril during five exhalations and inhalations. Then change over and close the right nostril for the same number. Continue in this way to the end of the group. This exercise is easy to practise.

Variation II. In this variation successive respirations take place through alternate nostrils. The difficulty lies in keeping the alternations synchronised with the respirations at speed. Proceed as follows:

> Exhale and inhale on the left (right nostril closed),
> Exhale and inhale on the right (left nostril closed),
> Exhale and inhale on the left (right nostril closed),
> Exhale and inhale on the right (left nostril closed), and so on

for the whole group.

Do not start Kapalabhati with alternate respiration before you have mastered the normal version. When the movement has become entirely automatic and your concentrated attention can be directed to the movements of the fingers, you can move on to this form of Kapalabhati. Start slowly and let the speed increase gradually by itself. All the other recommendations remain valid.

Effects of Kapalabhati
The principal effects of Kapalabhati are:

Rejection of residual air from the lungs. Even full yogic respiration does not completely empty the lungs of the last traces of stale air that remain at the end of an exhalation. However, the rapid succession of sharp expulsions in Kapalabhati gets rid of this residual air and thus constitutes a total cleansing of the lungs. It is an excellent preventive measure against tuberculosis.

Carbon dioxide (CO_2) Kapalabhati causes a substantial expulsion of carbon dioxide, whose level in the blood falls quickly. If the exercise is continued for two or three minutes, the whole organism is cleansed. This reduction of the carbon dioxide level in the organism is abnormal Kapalabhati but beneficial. Furthermore, the normal level is automatically reestablished soon after the end of the exercise. Logically speaking it would therefore seem that the exercise is pointless. The advantage is, however, that when the blood circulates slowly, the cells do not easily rid themselves of the carbon dioxide they produce. The temporary drop in the carbon dioxide level of the blood gives the cells the chance to eliminate their own carbon dioxide quickly.

Oxygen. At the same time as the blood cells lose carbon dioxide, they become saturated with oxygen. The resulting increase in cellular activity is particularly important for people who normally lead sedentary lives. Kapalabhati in this way stimulates cellular respiration, which produces a feeling of warmth throughout the body. Man in his natural state has sufficient physical exercise to ensure a good metabolism activity of the cells, but the civilised being, whose activity is slowed down, has a daily need for this extra oxygenation of the blood with its consequent increase in cellular respiration.

Blood circulation. I have several times drawn the reader's attention to the role of the diaphragm in activating the circulation of the blood. This role is even more important for the civilised being whose muscle contractions are much weaker than those of primitive man. Consequently, the return circulation of the venous blood, and with it the flow of arterial blood from the heart, is permanently slowed down. Kapalabhati transforms the diaphragm into a heavy-duty pump for the venous blood which is recycled and reoxygenated. Two or three minutes practising Kapalabhati causes all the tissues to vibrate. The whole organism trembles under the effect of Kapalabhati.

Adepts of Kundalini Yoga use the very prolonged practice of Kapalabhati to activate the centres of spiritual energy which correspond to the cosmic forces latent in ordinary man. This is why adepts who practise yoga with a spiritual aim, far from being excused the practice of Kapalabhati and other pranayama exercises, must practise them with more force and for longer than must those who only pursue a hygienic aim. In the West we might suppose the contrary to be true!

Kapalabhati produces an intense pranic activity in the organism, which is the reason why students who practise it for long periods are obliged to do so in the lotus posture. Reactions can be very violent and may result in the whole body shaking. For this reason the legs must be firmly locked in the lotus posture. It is evident that such intensive practice is only permissible under the supervision of an experienced guru. The danger is rather theoretical in the West, as these reactions only occur after practice so intense that it is beyond the reach of the Westerner, whose abdominal muscles would be exhausted long before the danger level was reached.

Lungs. Kapalabhati purifies the lungs and maintains the suppleness of the spongy tissue. The exchanges become more active.

Diaphragm. The diaphragm participates intensely though passively in Kapalabhati. It is not moved by the contraction of its own muscles but it is manipulated by the abdomen, which pushes the abdominal organs backwards and upwards against the diaphragm. In this way Kapalabhati maintains the mobility and suppleness of the diaphragm, the importance of which cannot be overestimated.

Abdomen. Kapalabhati causes an excellent control of all the muscles of the abdomen and particularly the large straight muscles which acquire the strength and suppleness so necessary to them. Moreover, the activity of the abdominal muscular belt tends to eliminate fatty deposits on the abdominal wall. Regular practice of Kapalabhati and other pranayama exercises causes oxidation and the disappearance of this undesirable fatty tissue.

Abdominal organs. All the organs of the abdominal cavity without exception are toned up and massaged. This applies to the digestive tract and associated glands. The digestion becomes more active and responsive, so that the sensation of heaviness after a meal is avoided.[*] Kapalabhati also activates intestinal peristalsis and fights both spastic and atonic constipation.

Nervous system. Kapalabhati has profound effects on the sympathetic nervous system in particular. The hyperoxygenation of the blood which is the normal excitant of the respiratory centre, combined with the reduction in carbon dioxide level, calms this centre and make its action felt throughout the sympathetic nervous system. Kapalabhati is an incomparable tonic for the entire nervous system.

---

[*] This does not mean that Kapalabhati should be practised just after a meal. On the contrary, this would disturb the digestion. The effect mentioned is thus indirect..

26 | The Effects of Kapalabhati on the Brain

In the preceding section on Kapalabhati we have studied the general repercussions of this fundamental pranayama exercise. These effects alone justify its regular practice, a powerful tonic to the whole system, as it increases the student's pranic potential. There is one point, however, that deserves separate study: the effects of Kapalabhati – and incidentally of all pranayama exercises – on the circulation of the blood and especially that in the brain.

A fact well known to physiologists but quite unknown to the general public is that respiration alters the volume of the brain. Most of us have some general idea of the brain, but we usually imagine it as enclosed within the skull, where it remains stationary like a nut in its shell. This comparison is often used because of the brain's resemblance to half a walnut. In fact, like a half-walnut, the brain is divided into two lobes and its surface has numerous convolutions. Although enclosed within the skull like a nut in its shell, the brain throbs and moves; its volume diminishes during inhalation as the lungs fill up with air and increases during exhalation. The variations in volume are proportional to the respiratory movement, for the brain behaves like a spongy mass, shrinking and enlarging according to the respiratory rhythm. This double movement influences the circulation of fluids in the brain, especially the blood. Because the brain is the greatest consumer of blood in the body, we realise how important is the circulation in this area.

Complete yogic breathing increases the volume change and thus favours the irrigation of the brain. Kapalabhati (and also Bhastrika) increase this flux enormously. Normal respiration decreases and increases the brain volume about eighteen times a minute, so imagine what happens when Kapalabhati involves 120 exhalations in the same time. This is real brain massage! It is accompanied by a pumping action of the arterial circulation, since on exhalation the brain fills with blood, and at the rate of 120 pump-strokes a minute a torrent of blood is forced into the brain, which is rinsed and irrigated. All the capillaries are opened up, and the cells of the brain and those of the endocrine glands enclosed in the brain, especially the very important pituitary and pineal glands, are invigorated. This is completely without danger as the pressure always stays within the normal physiological limits; only the circulation is accelerated. This Kapalabhati action effects a 'brain-washing' in the literal sense and the consequences are far-reaching. Irrigated by blood rich in oxygen, the brain benefits from a natural stimulation which for modern, sedentary man is most desirable. His normal superficial breathing is insufficient and the air he breathes is often stale and polluted.

The practice of yoga is so logical! While the asanas loosen all the joints of the body, stretch the muscles and free all the roots of the nerves, they prepare the organism to receive a supplement of prana without the risk of a 'prana short-circuit'. Accompanied by adequate respiration, the asanas increase the amount of prana in the human body and permit its harmonious distribution throughout the system. Pranayama adds its own effects and further increases the fixing and storage of prana in the appropriate accumulators (the chakras), whence it is distributed to all the organs that need it.

Pranayama stimulates the brain, the thinking organ, directly. It is cleansed of all its stagnant or sluggishly circulating blood and receives a flow of freshly oxygenated blood. If we remember that Kapalabhati means 'shining skull' or 'that which cleans the skull' (and its contents), we can readily believe that the real significance of the word is 'cleansing of the brain', which becomes lucid, alert and oxygenated. Thus irrigated, rinsed, stimulated and oxygenated, it is ready for the great adventure of exploring the mind. An amendable instrument, it will function efficiently during the practice of concentration. With a lucid brain there is much less risk of drowsiness, the most frequent interruptor of concentration exercises and meditation. Together with the acceleration of the blood circulation in the whole body, this stimulation of the brain and thereby of the central nervous system produces the special 'vibration' of the body that invigorates and tonifies every cell. The massage of the brain and the entire nervous system are the main effects of Kapalabhati. The change in brain volume also acts on the circulation of the cephalo-rachidian fluid.

In order to appreciate the tonic effect of Kapalabhati it is sufficient, after a tiring day, to practise it for three or four minutes (including rest periods) when the tiredness will at once disappear and you will feel ready to start work again. Fatigue and the resultant toxins are literally dissolved and swept away by the fresh blood which circulates at high speed in the brain. In a few minutes the brain cells recover their lost vitality and are again fresh and alert. This is why Kapalabhati acts as a pure and unique brain tonic.

During gymnastics also and in sporting activities it happens that the breathing accelerates after great physical effort, but this very effort almost immediately absorbs the extra oxygen which has been inhaled during accelerated respiration. During yoga, however, when the body remains motionless, muscular energy consumption is negligible and the oxygen and prana benefit the brain to the highest degree. This is why pranayama rests us and recharges our batteries while sport tires us, which is by no means a bad thing as we also need physical tiredness. Indeed modern man, who is almost wholly intellectual, ends up by making too great a demand on his brain and his nervous system. He needs an exercise like Kapalabhati to compensate.

We should practise Kapalabhati and, instead of living with a brain full of toxins, we shall then live dynamically but serenely with a 'shining skull', a purified and oxygenated brain. It is not surprising that the regular practice of Kapalabhati increases our powers of concentration, improves the memory and stimulates all the intellectual faculties.

27 | Bhastrika, the Bellows

In Indian villages the blacksmith is an important man. In his forge the bellows fan the charcoal which heats the iron. Bhastrika has taken its name from these bellows. It is a classical exercise but often misunderstood. Even the Gheranda Samhita (verses 75–6) is not very explicit:

'As the blacksmith's bellows dilate and contract continuously, so he [the yogi] inhales slowly through both nostrils while distending the abdomen; he then expels the air rapidly (when it makes the same noise as bellows). Having inhaled and exhaled twenty times, he must perform Kumbhaka (breath retention) and expel the air in the same way. The wise man will practise this Bhastrika-Kumbhaka three times. He will never suffer from illness but will always be in good health.'

This description might just as well apply to Kapalabhati. In fact Bhastrika has certain points in common with Kapalabhati. The two exercises are sometimes confused with one another, and certain teachers do not distinguish between them. However, if we study the various opinions and techniques we shall find that there are considerable differences. These are listed in the comparative table at the end of this section. Kapalabhati may be considered as an easier form of Bhastrika and consequently as a preparation for it.

Technique
The only postures allowed are siddhasana and the lotus. As a concession the student may use vajrasana at the beginning if he is incapable of holding either of the other two. When Bhastrika is practised, the entire respiratory apparatus goes into action. The basis of Bhastrika is the complete yogic respiration in three steps but practised with control of the abdominal belt.

Learning Bhastrika. Sit in the chosen posture and see that your spine stays straight and immobile during the whole exercise. Carry out yogic breathing as complete as possible with the abdomen controlled. Gradually accelerate the rhythm without reducing the volume of air inhaled.

It is very important that the acceleration be gradual so that volume is not sacrificed to speed (which should never exceed sixty breaths per minute). The slight constriction of the glottis (Ujjayi) produces a characteristic noise during Bhastrika.

The nostrils must be absolutely free during Bhastrika. Continue for about one minute regardless of the number of breaths taken during this time. Then hold your breath while carrying out the three Bandhas (Bandha Traya,* see p. 195). In the beginning you should not exceed forty forced exhalations. Slowly increase this to sixty so long as you can continue for at least a minute without fatigue. The inhalation preceding breath retention at the end must be as deep as possible. The breath should be held for as long as you can. At the end of the retention inhale a little air before exhaling *slowly* and completely through the *right* nostril (Pingala).

Interiorisation. During the retention in Bandha Traya concentrate on Muladhara Chakra. This is essential.

Bhastrika variation Bhastrika may also be practised as described above but with alternate breathing. Inhale through the left nostril (Ida), exhale through the right nostril (Pingala), re-inhale through Pingala, exhale through Ida, re-inhale through Ida and so on. At first go slowly in order to synchronise the movements of the hand that directs the alternation with the Bhastrika respiration. This variation is more powerful than ordinary Bhastrika, but it should not be attempted before normal Bhastrika has become spontaneous and comfortable. The respiration rate should not exceed fifty breaths per minute.

Physiological effects
Like all hyperventilation exercises, Bhastrika has deep repercussions throughout the system. It is very powerful and must be practised very carefully, especially at the beginning.

The blood becomes saturated with oxygen, while large quantities of carbon dioxide are expelled. The acidity of the blood and its carbon dioxide content are temporarily modified. Carbon dioxide is not a toxic gas; in a limited and stable amount it is a normal constituent of the blood. Persons in danger of suffocating will not be saved by administer-

---

* Bandha Traya, usually performed with empty lungs in order to ease and accentuate Uddiyana. The form of Bandha Traya described here is peculiar to Bhastrika.

ing oxygen but by carbon dioxide (although we do not yet know why carbon dioxide acts in this case as a rescuer). Normally only the excess carbon dioxide is eliminated as the blood passes through the cells of the lungs. The elimination of large amounts of carbon dioxide during Bhastrika (and also during Kapalabhati) lowers the blood's carbon dioxide level so in order to re-establish the normal level veryquickly the student must hold his breath with full lungs. In the meantime, however, cellular respiration has been accelerated by Bhastrika with a consequent revitalisation of the organism in the strictest sense of the word. For the other effects of Bhastrika the reader is referred to the section on Kapalabhati.

Pranic effects
Bhastrika is fundamental from the point of view of pranayama During the exercise the acceleration of the blood flow in the brain activates the resonating centres Ajna Chakra and Sahasrara Chakra. During breath retention the organs and resonating plexus of the lower chakras are activated. As already pointed out, concentration during retention must be on Muladhara Chakra. During Bhastrika there is a balance between Prana and Apana, which meet, and their union acts on Kapalabhati (stimulating the creative psychic centres in the human being). Furthermore, Bhastrika guides the pranic energy along Sushumna, the central conduit. The ascent of this energy is usually blocked by 'knots' (literal translation of granthis), but Bhastrika allows the energy developed by pranayama to continue its part through the 'knots' towards the centres leading to the level of individual integration in the brain, or rather its subtle counterpart Sahasrara. This pranayama is one of the best preparatory exercises fo Pratyahara (withdrawal of the senses) and for Dharana (concentration), which are the following stages of yoga.

Precautions
Bhastrika being one of the most powerful yoga exercises not only in itself but also by its acquisition of maximum breath retention with full lungs, it must be practised with common sense and without haste. I t can have bad effects on the heart, such as arhythmia (irregular beat) but these effects cease when the exercise stops; fortunately, therefore they are reversible. The lungs, however, can be affected be emphysema, which is not reversible.

In order to practise Bhastrika in complete safety, it must be done without violence. Speed must not be the principal objective and should not be confused with undue haste. If the practice is progressive, the lungs will become more elastic and be able to stand Bhastrika without damage, for we must remember that the air cells of the lungs are among the most delicate of body tissues. As far as the heart is concerned, Jalandhara Bandha, with its strong contraction of the neck muscles, guarantees safety. The table below sums up and compares the techniques of Kapalabhati and Bhastrika.

	Kapalabhati	Bhastrika
Type of respiration	Purely diaphragmatic and rather superficial with chest blocked (thrust far out).	Complete respiration (in three steps) with abdominal belt controlled, much deeper
Active parts	Abdomen.	Chest participates actively as does the whole respiratory system.
Inhalation/ exhalation ratio	Inhalation twice as long as exhalation. Stress on exhalation	
Maximum respiration rate	120 per minute	60 per minute.
Ujjayi	Very slight closure of the glottis.	
Power	Average.	Very powerful.
Effects	Cleans the respiratory tracts. Hyperventilation	The respiratory tracts must be free before the exercise is begun.
Interiorisation	Manipura Chakra.	Muladhara Chakra (during retention).

Ujjayi is one of the principal pranayamas, not only in itself but also because it is important in the practice of the asanas. This special application is dealt with at the end of the present section.

Whereas the etymology of Kapalabhati presents no difficulty, the interpretations of Ujjayi vary according to the author. Sometimes the word Ujjayi is split into a prefix *ud*, to lift up or to raise (cf. Ud-diyana Bandha), and *Jaya*, which is an ancient form of greeting in India (e.g. Jaya Ram). Thus Ujjayi is said to mean 'that which is expressed in a loud voice' because this pranayama is not silent. Others maintain that Ujjayi means 'that which leads to success' or 'the victorious', because the thorax is thrust out like the chest of a warrior. Perhaps both these explanations are correct since, by combing the noise with the expansion of the thorax, the two essential elements are united.

Technique
As a pranayama Ujjayi has two main forms, both of which are classical and complete. One of them is easier for the beginner. Before studying these two forms, remember that the characteristic element of Ujjayi rests in the partial blocking of the glottis so as to brake the incoming or outgoing air. Contract the muscles at the base of the neck near the collar-bone and inhale. The friction of the air thus checked causes a deep continuous noise which derives from neither the vocal chords nor the friction of the air against the soft palate as in snoring. The contraction of the glottis constricts the passages through which the air enters, the purpose of which is described under 'Effects' (p. 168). Inhalation and exhalation should both be moderately noisy and more or less at the same pitch. When breathing in Ujjayi' is instructed for the practice of certain asanas, it is this partial blocking of the glottis that is referred to.

Normal Ujjayi

Position. Ujjayi may be practised in all positions and under all circumstances when it accompanies the practice of asanas; in this case it means the partial closing of the glottis. When Ujjayi is regarded as a pranayama the posture required is either siddhasana, half-lotus or lotus, the last being preferable. Vajrasana is allowed only for beginners. The position of the arms is particularly important: they must be outstretched, with the backs of the hands against the knees and in Jnana Mudra, which means the mudra of the initiated (see following section).

Spine. The spine is in the correct position when the pelvis is slightly tilted forward. This is spontaneous in the lotus posture with both knees touching the ground so that the lumbar region is slightly hollow.

Inhalation (Puraka). Inhalation takes place with the abdomen controlled (see p. 103); it must be slow and mainly thoracic. When the diaphragm has descended enough to meet the growing resistance of the controlled abdominal belt, an effort must be made to take in as much air as possible by lifting and opening the ribs. Finally, the lungs must be completely filled by lifting the upper thorax. At the end of the inhalation it should be impossible to get any more air into the lungs. The chest is thrust forward so as to justify the name 'the victorious'. During the whole inhalation the glottis remains partially closed and the air produces the regular sound at constant pitch characteristic of Ujjayi. At the completion of inhalation the breath must be held by closing the glottis completely for two seconds – no more – and then exhaling.

Exhalation (Rechaka). Open the glottis slightly and contract the abdomen more vigorously. This starts exhalation, which must be accompanied by the same regular, uniform sound as inhalation. Then contract the thoracic muscles so as to bring the ribs together. When this has been achieved exhalation is completed by lowering the collar bones without bending forward. It is important to note that the spine stays absolutely straight and immobile during the whole exercise. The exhalation must last at least twice as long as the inhalation and the air must be expelled by the active contraction of the abdominal belt. At the end of the exhalation hold your breath for two seconds and then re-inhale as described above.

Interiorisation. During the whole exercise the student must concentrate on (a) the passage of air through the nostrils and particularly against their upper part, and (b) the noise of the air as it passes through the glottis (see 'Effects on the mind', below).

Duration. Cycles of at least ten respirations should be performed. After a rest, repeat the exercise for four or five cycles. Ujjayi should be practised daily for between five and ten minutes and should be followed by two or three minutes relaxation in Shavasana with normal breathing.

Purna- Ujjayi
Purna-Ujjayi is the most intensive form of this pranayama and must be reserved for students well advanced in the practice of yoga and experienced both in the normal form of Ujjayi and in breath retention. In fact, Purna-Ujjayi implies prolonged breath retention with full lungs.

Posture. Siddhasana (which may be made more comfortable without losing its effectiveness by placing a small pillow under the buttocks) or, preferably, it should be lotus. The left arm is in the same position as in simple Ujjayi with the hand in Jnana Mudra. The right arm, however, is bent so that the right hand can plug the nose for alternate respiration. The index and the middle finger are bent, the right thumb closes the right nostril, the ring finger and the little finger close the left nostril. This is the usual procedure, although some schools recommend placing the index and the middle finger at the root of the nose. Ujjayi should be practised throughout in Jalandhara Bandha although some yogis carry out Jalandhara Bandha only during breath retention (Kumbhaka).

Inhalation. Inhalation takes place through both nostrils. The right hand stays in place, ready to close the nostrils. The glottis is partly closed as in simple Ujjayi. The abdomen is controlled, and thoracic and subclavicular breathing is carried out as in simple Ujjayi. The facial muscles must be relaxed during inhalation and the braking of the air must always take place at the glottis and not in the nostrils, through which it must pass gently. (The air must not be projected against the mucous membrane.) Inhalation must always be as slow as in simple Ujjayi. I personally prefer to practise Jalandhara Bandha during all phases.

Retention (Kumbhaka). Breath retention, which in simple Ujjayi is only symbolic, is an essential element of this exercise and Jalandhara Bandha is compulsory during this phase. This Jalandhara must be very energetic, i.e. the contraction of the neck muscles must be strong enough to block the respiratory tracts completely. The nose is closed by the fingers. Breath retention must last as long as is consistent with the general rules for retention. The thorax must stay expanded. During retention the abdomen should be pulled in, so as to push the viscera towards the spine, thus further increasing the intra-abdominal pressure. It is essential that Kumbhaka be accompanied by Mula Bandha.

Exhalation (Rechaka). Hold the breath until a slight vibration in the region of the solar plexus is felt, but no longer. Exhalation takes place through the left nostril exclusively. Exhalation should be prolonged as much as possible and last at least twice as long as inhalation. Progressive training will lead to a duration four times that of inhalation, which is the ultimate objective, not to be achieved in a hurry. Inhalation is correct when the Ujjayi sound remains continuous and at the same pitch. Exhalation should be as complete as possible and even forced.

Re-inhale after a short retention and two or three seconds with empty lungs. This new inhalation is a test. It is not sufficient to block the breath comfortably and then to exhale freely and slowly; you must also be able to re-inhale in the same controlled way as in simple Ujjayi. If, after a retention followed by a slow exhalation, you are forced to re-inhale hurriedly, you have overdone the retention and you must reduce the duration of Khumbaka until you are able to continue the whole Purna-Ujjayi cycle without discomfort. If occasionally your respiratory capacity is exceeded, this is not important provided it does not become habitual, when it could cause heart and lung trouble (see 'Counter-indications').

Interiorisation. As in simple Ujjayi.

Duration. In India 'full-time' yogis perform from 250 to 300 cycles. With an average retention this means at least the same number of minutes. Thus Ujjayi is performed for four hours or more at a time, but it is clear that this would be impossible for a Westerner who, to begin with, will find a series of from five to twenty Ujjayi quite enough. This can be increased gradually to fifteen to twenty minutes, which would not be bad.

Counter-indications
Persons suffering from heart or lung trouble should avoid all pranayama exercises with long breath retention. But if Ujjayi without retention (simple Ujjayi) is practised while lying down with the legs raised, it will benefit the heart; for people in good health Ujjayi is a wonderful heart exercise.

Effects
Yoga is the only discipline which tries to create considerable pressure changes in the abdomen and in the lungs. Uddiyana Bandha, Nauli and breathing with control of the abdomen considerably alter the pressures within the body. Only these exercises can reduce abdominal and thoracic pressure in a controlled way. Air inhaled normally penetrates the lungs only because of a reduction in thoracic pressure, although this reduction is slight. In the same way, in exhalation air leaves the lungs through a relaxation of the intercostal muscles, perhaps helped by contraction of the abdominal muscles, causing an excess pressure in the lungs. The rib-cage acts like the bellows of a forge. This comparison will help us to understand the reason for the partial constriction of the glottis. If we reduce the opening of the bellows and yet allow to pass the same amount of air in the same time, we need more energy (a greater pressure reduction) and during exhalation we have to press harder to expel the air. The partial constriction of the glottis acts in the same way and gives a greater reduction in intra-thoracic pressure during inhalation, which considerably increases the suction effect exerted on the venous circulation by the lungs. The effects of respiration with control of the abdomen are greatly increased by Ujjayi. The pressure in the lungs increases during exhalation and thereby helps to maintain their elasticity.

The gaseous and pranic exchanges are improved in Ujjayi as compared with ordinary breathing or even yogic respiration with abdominal control. Compression of the abdominal organs stimulates the psychic energy centres related to the lower abdomen, notably Manipura Chakra and Svadisthana Chakra. The practice of Mula Bandha, indispensable for the protection of the lower pelvis against excess intra-abdominal pressure, also acts on Mulandhara Chakra.

Effects on the mind
In Ujjayi, and especially in Purna-Ujjayi, the reciprocal interpen-

etration of Hatha Yoga and Raja Yoga becomes evident. The mental interiorisation which develops when the attention is focused on the passage of air through the nostrils and on the continuous sound produced has the effect of absorbing the mind completely and of reducing useless intellectual activity to a minimum. A very slight Ujjayi is a great help for starting meditation. The practice of Ujjayi awakens pranic and psychic energies. Jalandhara Bandha adds its own effects when it accompanies Purna-Ujjayi.

Ujjayi during the asanas
A characteristic of yoga as practised in the south of India is the introduction of Ujjayi in the practice of the asanas and sun worship. The partial closure of the glottis and the characteristic noise of Ujjayi are continued during the whole session. The breath is never held at any moment; it comes and goes continuously at the level of the glottis. Inhalation and exhalation are always of the same duration in order to balance prana and apana, which is extremely important. Sometimes the rhythm increases, particularly at the peak of an asana. For instance, during the dynamic phase of the Cobra, breathing is balanced in Ujjayi but rather slow. As the posture becomes more advanced, breathing tends to accelerate of its own accord. The same happens during sun worship. The student should not resist this tendency but rather encourage it. Ujjayi can also be practised while walking and even while running.

29 | Jnana Mudra, the Gesture of the Initiate

The gesture of the initiate is a symbolic gesture accompanying meditation and certain pranayamas. The palms of the hands are turned upwards; the fingers and thumbs are stretched. The index fingers are then bent inwards and the thumbs are bent to meet them. The nails of the index fingers are placed in the creases of the thumb joints, while the other fingers remain stretched and together. The union of the thumb and the index finger has a symbolic value, for the thumb represents the I or self, especially its human expression, since the thumb is the most 'human' of all and no animal has one. It is the opposition of the thumb to the other fingers that distinguishes a hand from a paw, all of whose digits face the same way. The hand is thus a creative instrument able to give shape to crude matter and provide it with a reflection of man's intelligence. Without the help of the thumb, the other fingers would be powerless to carry out the least human work.

In order to fulfil its role the thumb is placed apart from the fingers and in opposition. It watches them and judges them, but is always ready to co-operate. When fingerprints are taken it is the thumb which is most significant.

The index finger
This is the finger of individualisation. It symbolises the little individual ego. As its name implies, it is the pointer. The thumb is the symbol of the I and the index finger that of the ego.

The meeting of the index finger with the thumb
The other fingers represent various aspects of the human being and different schools have different interpretations of their symbolism. Thus the ring finger, which carries the symbol of marriage, is sometimes said to symbolise our attachment to sensual pleasures. The middle finger is then the symbol of rajasic ambition and so on. However, the essential element in the symbolism of Jnana Mudra is the joining of the thumb and the index finger. (The idea of union, of bringing together that which was previously separated, recurs constantly in yoga.) The index finger (the ego) has to leave the other fingers and move towards the

thumb (the I) which itself moves towards the index finger. Their union creates a closed ring, the symbol of the infinite. The union of index finger and thumb thus symbolises the cosmic integration of the I with the ego.

30 | Sitkari, Sitali and Plavini

These three pranayamas are minor exercises compared with those studied so far. Their practical applications in the West are very limited, mainly because of the climate. They are mentioned here only for the sake of completeness.

Sitkari – Sitali

Sitkari and Sitali include breathing through the mouth, which is supposed to be refreshing and is obviously useful in tropical climates. They are also supposed to combat thirst and are important for students living in India. In our damp western climate there is little to recommend breathing through the mouth, as the air entering the lungs needs first to be warmed and conditioned by its passage through the nose. Prolonged practice of these exercises could cause sore throat or bronchitis.

Shramari

This is a breathing exercise accompanied by a characteristic sound. It is difficult to describe clearly how it should be practised.

Plavini

Plavini – the float – is a minor pranayama. The student swallows air through the mouth and the gullet so that the stomach distends like a balloon and sounds hollow when tapped. The student can then float indefinitely in water, hence its name – the float. In the West it is difficult to imagine a practical or pranic use for this exercise.

Part 3

ESOTERIC PRANAYAMA,
ITS BASES AND ITS PRACTICE

So far we have made no distinction between Prana, the cosmic energy in all its forms in the universe around us, and prana, the energy which penetrates us, accumulates in us, circulates and emerges again, because that prana working within us is simply a temporary specialisation of universal cosmic energy. Similarly, there is no chemical difference between the water which covers three-quarters of the globe as oceans, which drips from the roofs as rain, which we absorb in our food and drink, and the water which constitutes three-quarters of the weight of our body. Water goes through a planetary cycle: it evaporates from the ocean, forms clouds in the sky, falls as rain, animates living matter (there is no life without water) then flows into rivers and returns to the ocean whence it came. However, as soon as water enters the body we give it a different name according to its internal function. When absorbed by the digestive tract it becomes blood which actually is mainly water with red corpuscles, white corpuscles and other components. The original water also changes into lymph, interstitial liquid in which our cells are immersed, and intracellular liquid.

Similarly, cosmic Prana penetrates our body and forms our pranic, our energising body. It is the pranic body which animates the crude and dense matter and forms our tangible and visible body. For yogis, just as water is 'specialised', so prana is diversified in the pranic body and changes its name. The whole vital energy which animates the material body becomes breath, or pneuma; in Sanskrit *Vayu*, which literally means 'air'. Vayu, the vital breath, assures the various functions of the body. In opposition to the dense, physical body which is subdivided into distinct anatomical structures, the pranic body forms an indivisible entity, differentiated only in its vital activities or particular functions, which are not rigidly localised in any definite part of the body. The function creates the corresponding organ and animates it.

Just as the dense body must be fed, must take from the outside world the material elements which compose it, the pranic body must also appropriate some prana from the outside world. This appropriation of energy is called Prana-Vayu. Prana-Vayu includes all the subtle prana-absorption mechanisms. Its essential organ is the respiratory system. It is situated mainly in the thorax although there are other ways of penetration such as through the tongue and the skin. The absorption of liquid or solid food depends also on Prana-Vayu. Energy is then assimilated. All assimilation functions of our dense body are directed by a certain form of energy called Samana-Vayu. This specialised function of prana digests our food, assimilates it, leads it to the various organs. Its principal centre is between the diaphragm and the navel. Next, energy must be distributed and set in motion wherever the need is felt. This function is performed by Vyana-Vayu, whose action is much more diffuse than those already mentioned, as it pervades the entire body. It ensures blood and lymph circulation as well as the circulation of energy along the nerves. In contrast to inanimate objects, one of the characteristics of life is that it is a dynamic process, a constant flow of physical particles as well as electromagnetic energising currents, and perhaps of other forms of energy which are still to be discovered. Life is a river whose shores (our bodies) are fairly stable but the water is never the same!

However, it is not enough to assimilate energy and matter. They must also be eliminated. The function of elimination is ensured by Apana-Vayu. Prana-Vayu and Apana-Vayu are the most important pranas in the body. All functions of excretion depend on Apana-Vayu whose action is oriented downwards and outwards. It is Apana-Vayu which animates the kidneys, filters the urine, releases the sphincters during urination and empties the bladder. It is Apana which directs the stool towards the rectum and, at the required moment, releases the anal sphincter and expels waste matter. Apana-Vayu releases the menses, discharges the sperm. Apana-Vayu functions during childbirth. The Apana is situated more particularly in the lower abdomen (sub-umbilical area) and deals mainly with the pelvic and sexual organs. But its role does not end there; it is also Apana-Vayu that eliminates excess water as perspiration. Finally, it expels gas residues through the respiratory tracts.

The lungs have thus a dual pranic function. First, they are the seal of Prana-Vayu, with all the air ducts ranging from the nose to the air cells of the lungs, since they serve mostly to collect the outer prana Besides, the lungs constitute an important outlet. During exhalation when we breathe out carbon dioxide and other waste products in the form of gas, this is the work of Apana-Vayu. Other Vayus are active in our bodies and the energy anatomy of the yogis is as complex as our descriptive anatomy!

The last of the main Vayus is Udana-Vayu, situated in the throat.

Its function is expression, because human beings express themselve mostly by speaking. It is Udana-Vayu which enables thought to express itself, regulates the air supply and the tension of the vocal cords when we speak. Other accessory Vayus (or Pranas) have very special functions, such as sneezing (Devadatta), yawning (Krikal) blinking (Kurma), etc. In whatever form it may be and in whatever part of the body it may occur, the absorption of prana is the work of Prana-Vayu which constitutes the 'entrance' pole. Whatever comes out of the organism, wherever it may be and in whatever form, is controlled by Apana-Vayu. There must be an equilibrium between the two: our health depends on it. Constipation, malfunctioning of the kidneys, insufficient elimination of carbon dioxide by the lungs, and lack of permeability of the pores are the main causes of illness. Should any of these functions stop entirely, a most serious crisis would ensure When the kidneys cease to function, death from uremia follows! Apana-Vayu is as vital as Prana-Vayu. The 'exit' pole must balance the 'entrance' pole. We understand now why yogis, especially in the south of India, attach great importance to the equilibrium between inhalation and exhalation during the practice of asanas.* Between the two poles the inner circuits are situated on various levels: assimilation = Samana: distribution = Vyana; expression = Udana. They are very important too, but from a practical viewpoint they are more difficult to control than the 'entrance' and 'exit' poles. The balanced functioning of Prana-Vayu and Apana-Vayu conditions and ensures the correct functioning of assimilation and energy circulation almost automatically. The balancing action of Apana is essential. It takes place mostly below the navel. Asvini Mudra and Mula Bandha** enable you to gain conscious and voluntary control of these forces. But equilibrium between these two poles is not the only goal that yogis try to reach: during pranayama they strive to reverse the direction of the flow of Apana energy, which is usually downwards, in order to draw upwards to meet Prana-Vayu. The union of Prana-Vayu and Apana Vayu gives results which are considered very important for the ultimate yoga experience.

---

   *   See *Je perfectionne mon Yoga*, p. 14.
  **   See Sections 34 and 35, pp. 186–194

THE FIVE PRINCIPAL MODIFICATIONS OF PRANA (VAYUS)

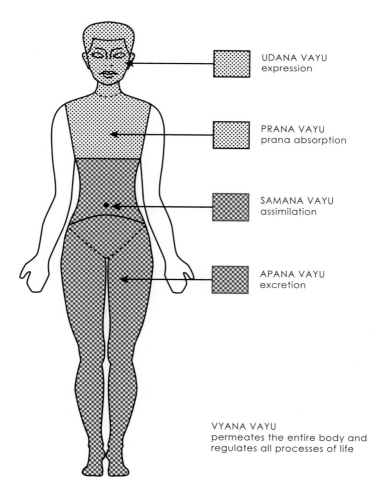

UDANA VAYU
expression

PRANA VAYU
prana absorption

SAMANA VAYU
assimilation

APANA VAYU
excretion

VYANA VAYU
permeates the entire body and
regulates all processes of life

3 2 | S u r y a   B h e d a   K u m b h a k a

The value and meaning of Surya Bheda Kumbhaka can only be appreciated if the notions of Prana-Vayu and Apana-Vayu and the importance of their equilibrium are properly understood. The yogi tries to unite and control them, and in this connection Surya Bheda Kumbhaka is a remarkable exercise. Yet what are the meaning and derivation of these words? Surya (the sun) has become familiar to us thanks to Surya-Namaskar, the sun worship that yogis perform at sunrise. Thus it is the solar (right) nostril - Pingala - which is referred to here. Bheda means 'that which pierces'. Thus the purpose of the exercise is 'to pierce' the solar nadi, to make it permeable. Many texts refer to this exercise simply as 'Surya Bhodana' and omit the word 'Kumbhaka', but it is useful, at least in the title, to give the complete name, since the characteristic of this exercise is prolonged breath retention. In fact, Suryabheda is a special form of breath retention.

Position
Any position other than the lotus or the siddhasana is excluded. Vajrasana is tolerated. The hand is placed as for alternate breathing, since the nostrils will be closed (turn and turn about*). In Suryabheda inhalation is *always* performed through the solar (right) nostril. Inhale as deeply as possible with abdominal control, then close both nostrils, and hold your breath in Jalandhara Bandha. At the end of breath retention, when it becomes uncomfortable or just before exhaling, draw in the abdomen as much as possible (Uddiyana Bandha), trying to push the organs back toward the spine. Do Mula Bandha at the same time. In a way, it is Bandha Traya but it takes place only at the very end of breath retention. Do Jalandhara with maximum contraction. When retention becomes uncomfortable, exhale slowly through the lunar or left nostril (Ida). Do not pause but immediately start a new inhalation through the right nostril and repeat the process. To be on the safe side, you should remain capable of exhaling slowly, immediately resuming the exercise without having to take normal breaths between

---

*   See Section 12, pp. 66–71

two Suryabhedas. If exhalation is not controlled and there is need to catch your breath between two retentions, you have gone beyond your capability. If this happens only once, it is not serious: you just turn back and hold your breath for a shorter time. It would be dangerous to go regularly beyond your capability.

Yogis carry this exercise very far. They hold their breath until perspiration shows at the root of their hair and on their nails. Western students would be well advised not to emulate them, first because they go a long way beyond what is considered safe practice, and secondly because perspiration starts much more readily in India than in the West. It is preferable to practise longer and safely rather than risk pulmonary or cardiac troubles.

Effects
Gheranda Samhita declares that 'Surya Bheda Kumbhaka counteracts degeneration and death; it awakens Kundalini and increases the "body's fire". That "fire" is cellular breathing, evidenced by a feeling of warmth first in the cheeks, then in the whole body, and by a stimulation of digestion ["digestive fire"].' Hatha Yoga Pradikipa adds: 'By this process, air is directed forcibly into Sushumna.' Consequently this exercise gives prana control in the human body, the penetration of the solar nadi making it permeable, while Bandha Traya and Kumbhaka awaken latent energy and open up the Sushumna nadi .

We shall not dwell too much on these subtle repercussions but this pranayama constitutes a general tonic for the body and reinforces the vitality and psychic tonus, although its practice should be restricted to advanced students, especially when long retention is involved. This exercise should not be performed too close to bedtime. The best time is in the morning or at noon, before eating. Naturally, it should never be performed immediately after a meal. However, if retention is really short, all students including beginners, may practise it profitably.

Summary
Inhale slowly through Pingala (right nostril). Retention with full lungs (with Bandha Traya) prolonged to the utmost. Exhale slowly through Ida (left nostril) and repeat. On an average, a series of five is sufficient for Westerners.

3 3 | K u n d a l i n i

The individual and the species poles

For each individual the moment of truth occurs when the paternal sperm penetrates the ovum and fertilises it. There are millions of sperms at the start of the great race for the survival of the species, though only a few come close to the ovum that awaits them. The winner of the race enters the ovum and the ovum closes around it, and at that moment the first complete cell of a new individual is formed.

For you or for me to be here today an incalculable number of 'chances' took place. Had any other sperm penetrated the ovum it would not have been quite you or I who would have been born. If our fathers had married other women other human beings would have taken our names and might have been born at the same time, but they would not be us. Even supposing our fathers had married our mothers but had been away at the time when we were in fact conceived, the ova which gave origin to you and me would not have been fertilised and we would not be here discussing this subject. It was the same for our paternal and maternal grandparents and so on back to the origin of the human species. What an incredible sequence of 'chances' occurred for either of us to be living now!

From the moment the sperms entered the ova the dice were cast. We were there whole, carrying the hereditary capital of the species and an enormous sum of potentials. We have so far succeeded in showing only a small number of these; many others will remain latent.

The fertilised cell is the union of half the paternal and half the maternal genetic capital. At the beginning a human being is unicellular, but not for long. This single cell will soon be polarised under the impulse of the vital dynamism of the mother cell (the fertilised ovum), the first complete cell of his individuality. The essential elements of the nucleus will separate and move towards the poles of the cell, which will split into two; this is the first mitosis. Then things happen fast. The two cells become four, eight, sixteen and so on. The vital dynamism of cellular multiplication will continue for years at a pace which our minds cannot imagine, and yet the mind itself is composed of millions of these cells which are all descended from the original one.

Let us return to the moment when we were formed of four cells only, for an essential differentiation is about to take place: three of those cells will multiply very rapidly and by successive stages develop into the three large cell groups. The first group is the *ectoderm* which will become the skin and the nervous system. It will be our frontier guard and our 'public relations' service and also 'the executives', the nerve cells which will govern our whole inner and social life. Another cell will multiply to create our skeleton, cover it with the voluntary muscles and form vessels – arteries, capillaries, veins – and will fill it with blood; this is the *mesoderm* . A third cell will produce the respiratory system (larynx, bronchi, lungs and their smaller branches), plus the whole digestive tract with its glands (liver, pancreas, etc.); this is the *endoderm*. But what about the fourth cell? While its sisters are multiplying at high speed, the fourth reproduces much more slowly. Soon it will be covered and enveloped with formations coming from the three other cells. It gives birth to the genital system. It is the enclave of the species which, through it, seeks to safeguard the future. Indeed, the sexual cells represent a charter of all the body cells. Until puberty and adulthood they remain in the background while the 'individual' cells multiply endlessly. When the individual is an adult, their multiplying power slows down while the sexual cells multiply. The sexual cells form the enclave of the species, the 'species' pole situated in the pelvis, in the sacral area. As for the 'individual' pole, it is placed at the opposite end, in the skull, in the brain where individualised thinking originates. The spine is the vital axis and the link between the two poles.

The reserve cells represent the immortality of the species within us, since the sexual cells escape death when they leave the body to join another half and form a new mother cell which will give birth to a new individual. Only the descendants of the first three cells, the somatic cells, will die. Throughout our lives there will be an activity and a continuous interaction between these two poles. In the 'individual' pole, in the brain, the pituitary gland acts on the genital organs and controls their development during the whole of our youth. The 'species' pole acts on all body functions through its male or female hormones, determines the shape of our body (secondary sexual characteristics) and even acts on our psyche. A balanced interaction between the two poles is essential. The immortal dynamism of the species, which is the motive power of evolution throughout the generations, is situated at the base of the spine. This cosmic dynamism, which contains all the latent energy for the future evolution of the species and which also contains its past and controls its present, is undoubtedly Kundalini. These potentials for personal and genetic evolution, hence for evolution of the species, are dormant within each human being. The ambition of pranayama in its highest form is to awaken this dynamism.

For the species the individual is everything and nothing; in order to exist, the species must be carried and represented by individuals. Without individuals there is no species. On the other hand, the individual is unimportant to the species; for the immortal species (at least as immortal as one can be on this earthly manifestation level, since this planet will return to the nothingness whence it came) not only is the death of individuals an incident of no importance, it is the very condition for its evolution. In fact, it is because individuals are mortal that the species can replace them with others and can consequently evolve. The death of individuals makes evolution possible because it guarantees the plasticity of the species. Here we have a paradoxical situation in that, in order to survive, the species gives every individual an intense desire to live: all other instincts of man (or rather of individuals, since this applies to all species) proceed from the instinct to live or to survive. That is why we all wish to live as long as possible and why death frightens those who do not grasp its profound meaning. In order to evolve, the species must eliminate individuals after a certain length of time.

Let us take the case of the lemmings, small rodents similar to field mice. For two, three, sometimes four years, they lead an unexceptional existence in their holes, eat and reproduce, but like other rodents they have an enormous reproductive capacity. Then suddenly, as if called by a radio signal, they leave their burrows in swarms; as in a perfectly organised migration they form hundreds of lines and, just as rivulets join into streams and swell the rivers that eventually flow into the sea, so hundreds of thousands of lemmings form innumerable troops crossing everything on their way in their *Drang nach dem Westen*. They cross fields, forests, streams and rivers, even cities! What is especially remarkable is that this should take place with these individuals simultaneously, even at a great distance from one another. Eventually they reach the sea but even this does not stop them! The river of lemmings flows into the sea, and the sea is soon covered with rodents swimming westward. Quickly exhausted, they drown in millions, and their bodies are cast back by the tide to accumulate on the shore.

Some scientists have tried to explain this strange behaviour as an atavistic migration memory of the species deriving from remote times, and from this they have sought to prove their theory of continental drift. Unfortunately for the proponents of this theory, the lemming species was created only during the tertiary era and at that time the continents were already at about the same distance from each other as they are today, that is, thousands of kilometres apart. But biologists have solved this mystery: this mass suicide occurs when the overpopulated territory will no longer permit the species to survive. Threatened with extinction, it prefers to sacrifice millions of individuals for the benefit of a small number which remain on solid ground and reproduce, thus ensuring the continuity of the species.

The species may be considered as an integration level comprising the individuals and capable of acting on them. The species is not a myth but rather a dynamic force present in each individual yet surpassing him. Another element should be added: the species has been polarised at a different level and shows two complementary aspects, the Absolute Feminine and the Absolute Masculine aspects, which are reflected with relative perfection in every individual. That polarisation is fundamental: all species except unicellular species have sex, and sex is one of the cosmic aspects of life. It pervades the entire individual, his body as well as his mind, and affects his whole behaviour. When Freud declared that everything is libido, he meant we are steeped in sex, which determines our relationships with other individuals of our own species or with other species, or even with inanimate objects. The 'sex' concept is not, therefore, limited to the genitals, as is too often believed. Obviously we have genitals corresponding to our sex, but there is much more to it than that. It is a way of being. Nor is sexual relationship limited to the sexual act. In most people's minds, to have sexual relations is synonymous with mating, but this is a serious confusion. When Freud states that a newborn child has sexual relations with its mother, he means the behaviour of the newborn child is already determined by its sex: a male infant behaves differently towards his mother than he does towards his father, brother or sister. To stretch the point, one might say we have sexual relations even with objects: a man does not drive his car as a woman does! If 'sexual relation' refers to any form of behaviour influenced by the sex of the individual, we might say we have sexual relations with all men and all women. Yet it still remains that polarisation is best expressed in the sexual organs. When the Absolute Feminine aspect in one individual meets the Absolute Masculine aspect in another individual and together they form a couple, even temporarily, it is a cosmic event for the species. Sexuality is the motive power of the individual and the basic dynamism of the species. The individual and the species find fulfilment in the sexual act. To transpose sexuality on a cosmic level is the only way of bestowing on it a sacred character in the absolute sense of the word.

As far as sexuality is concerned, humanity fluctuates between various attitudes: (1) a taboo which leads to inhibition through excessive puritanism; (2) a 'healthy sexuality', aiming at a 'normal' satisfaction of a normal need without any rigid moral obstacles as in any other body functions; (3) a 'sublimation' which can only be an exceptional happening, and (4) a 'cosmisation' (if I am allowed to create a new word) which includes the 'healthy' satisfaction while at the same time exceeding it. This last aspect is characteristic of yoga. This 'cosmisation' is the basis of secret tantric practices, probably the oldest form of yoga, native to ancient India. Modern yoga may be the result of an interaction between the concepts brought by the Aryan invaders and some prehistoric notions from the Dravidian aborigines, in particular Ha-Tha Yoga, Yoga of the sun (*Ha*) and of the moon (*Tha*), Yoga of the masculine and feminine polarisation, Yoga of Ida and Pingala polarisation, Yoga of the 'species–individual' polarisation. That is why tantrism includes ritual sexual practices which it would be pointless to deny, but their purpose was to make all sexuality sacred. Is it purely coincidental that the base of the spine should be called the 'sacrum'?

The activation of the 'species' pole is one of the essential elements of pranayama, since our life comes from the very dynamism of the species. The practice of Mula Bandha and of Asvini Mudra aims at controlling the species pole and creating a flow between this sacred pole and the individual pole in the brain, the thousand-petalled lotus, the highest chakra (in the individual sense). When the forces of the species ascend the spine to join with the forces of the individual, this constitutes a cosmic event too. The dynamism of the species – that which caused and controlled the evolution of the human race over millions of years – is within us, very active until adulthood, then becomes dormant, latent, as Kundalini. That is why Kundalini is represented as a serpent, symbolising the strength of the species, coiling itself three and a half times around the lingam, the sign of Shiva, the sacred phallus represented inside a triangle pointing downwards, symbol of the female sex. Kundalini is not sexuality or the meeting of the sexes: if it were, yogis would have been satisfied with representing the lingam inside a triangle pointing downwards and no more. Therefore Kundalini is linked to sexuality, expressing itself through sexuality but not identical with it. Besides, the whole of Hindu mythology is but a symbolic representation of the cosmic forces! Shiva is the male cosmic principle and Shakti is its female complement, and from their union species are born. Shakti symbolises primordial nature.

Returning to the 'species' and 'individual' poles within us, it is through a conscious control of the perineum, through Mula Bandha and Asvini Mudra in particular, that the individual can mobilise and awaken the latent forces of the species and use them 'creatively' within himself as a factor of individual evolution. Because of descriptions given in some books, yoga adepts often imagine that the awakening of Kundalini is as sudden and as explosive as an atomic chain reaction and that it occurs without transition. In a sense they are right, since Kundalini can awaken in a spectacular manner and transmute the whole human being. But that awakening can be achieved only after years of effort, thanks to the knowledge and practice of secret techniques under the personal and continuous supervision of a guru. These cases are extremely rare, and as far as I know there is no authenticated case today. On the other hand, a certain intensification of the normal current between species and individual may very well be realised. Whereas a total awakening of Kundalini may be very dangerous (let me reassure you, it is impossible to arrive at this point 'accidentally' through practices described in this or other books), a partial and gradual awakening is harmless because it can be controlled by anyone applying yoga techniques. No explosion, not even a short-circuit should be anticipated. A person who practises pranayama together with bandhas, is certain not only to control the pranic energy which penetrates him, to become capable of accumulating and directing it at will, he can also benefit from the basic vital dynamism which is represented within him by the genital pole and develop his real 'creativity'.

The practice of pranayama cannot be disassociated from that of mudras and bandhas. When pranayama leads to any disturbance of physical or mental health, it is usually either because the student practises pranayama without submitting to the discipline of asanas, or because he follows some theoretical or fragmentary instruction he has picked up haphazardly, especially without integrating mudras and bandhas with pranayama. Mudras and bandhas serve to control and guide the psychic and pranic forces engendered or set in motion. To practise pranayama without bandhas can be as disastrous as sending an electric current into a circuit without transformers or fuses; localised short-circuits, which would be absolutely harmless if the network were normally protected, can put the whole network into short-circuit and cause incalculable damage. Some well-intentioned but ill-informed students thus create pranic short-circuits in their bodies.

Jalandhara Bandha is already familiar to us, and so is Udiyyana Bandha. We shall now add two exercises which have so much in common that they must be studied together: Asvini Mudra and Mula Bandha. To understand their importance and purpose and to use them properly it is indispensable to make a brief excursion into the fields of anatomy and physiology.

In the practice of pranayama the yogi applies pressure and releases it in the trunk at the thoracic level (above the diaphragm) and at the abdominal level. In breathing with abdominal control there is a struggle between the muscles which lower the diaphragm and push the organs downwards and forwards and the contracted abdominal wall which resists that pressure instead of yielding to it. The result is an increase in intra-abdominal pressure with all its beneficial effects.

The abdomen may be compared to a saucepan. On top is the lid (mobile), the dome of the diaphragm. The saucepan's sides are the abdominal wall, the back and side muscles and the spine; its bottom is the pelvis. If you look at a picture of the pelvis you will see that the bottom of this basin-shaped cavity is in fact pierced, but the aperture is closed by several important muscles and ligaments which form the pelvic floor. Now imagine pressing on the contents with the lid; the pressure will be distributed in all directions, both horizontally towards the walls and downward towards the base. The horizontal pressure is firmly retained by the controlled abdomen, but from the pressure exerted on the base, on the pelvic bones, there is nothing to fear, as they can stand any physiological pressure. But the bottom of the pelvis, the pelvic floor, is soft and relaxed and will yield to the pressure from above. It must therefore be controlled too; in other words it must be contracted and strengthened. This is done by Mula Bandha and Asvini Mudra.

The pelvic floor is composed mainly of the muscles which lift the anus (Levatores Ani) and of the coccyx muscles (Coccygei). They close up the aperture in the lower pelvis and are firmly hung between the pubic symphysis, the coccyx and the sacrum. It is like a hammock of muscles stretched between the various bones of the pelvis. This hammock also has openings for the genital organs and the anus and these openings are the weak points. To ensure the strength of the whole hammock (the muscles representing its fabric), it is reinforced by a net made of a very resilient layer of fibres. By contracting these muscles, Mula Bandha and Asvini Mudra enable the hammock to resist the increased pressure from the organs which are pushing down the diaphragm. Things are actually more complicated than that; there are also many important muscles and some vital nervous centres in this area, but the explanation given above will suffice for our purpose.

Asvini Mudra

We shall now study and practise Asvini Mudra, the manipulation of the anal sphincter and the contraction of the muscles on the pelvic floor which is the central element of Mula Bandha. Asvini Mudra makes you conscious of this area, strengthens its muscles and makes later practice of Mula Bandha possible without difficulty.

Etymology

Asvini means 'mare' in Sanskrit. In other words this Mudra is 'the Mudra of the Mare'. The name has a simple explanation. After expelling its stools a mare dilates and contracts its anus several times: Asvini Mudra imitates this and makes the anal sphincter work. All day long this sphincter keeps the lower orifice of the digestive tract, the anus, closed, and like all sphincters remains contracted continuously except when it is necessary to evacuate the faeces. This is the normal situation, but the anal sphincter and the muscles around it may be faced with less normal circumstances. Suppose circumstances prevent you from having a bowel movement just when you receive a call; you can resist the urge. But a baby cannot do so because it cannot yet control this muscle consciously. What a baby cannot do you can. The more pressing the urge, the more firmly and wilfully you must contract the anal sphincter and all the area in the region of the perineum. In yoga language this contraction is called 'Acuncana'.

The reverse circumstance is possible too: constipation, which will, in fact, not trouble you if you practise your asanas regularly and if your diet is right. But in constipation, when internal pressure is used, the sphincter will often open but without result, except that the anus protrudes from the perineum. This condition is called 'Prakashana'. Asvini Mudra is the practice of combining Acuncana and Prakashana in alternation: first a strong contraction of the anal sphincter and of the muscles which lift the anus, then a thrust to push the anus down by relaxing the sphincter. The repeated alternation of this process without interruption is Asvini Mudra.

Rhythm. A three-second contraction followed by a three-second relaxation.

Series. Start with a series of five, then gradually increase the number.

Posture
Asvini Mudra may be performed in any posture, but certain postures are recommended when practising Asvini Mudra as a separate exercise.

On the back. Lie down on your back and bend your knees so that your back is perfectly flat with feet about 30 cm apart. In this position it is much easier to make the anal sphincter work because the abdominal wall can be relaxed very easily. Practise for five minutes, then relax.

Combined with asanas. Asvini Mudra may also be practised in Sarvangasama. Lie down in the classical Sarvangasama posture, then bend your knees slightly and keep them apart. Asvini is particularly helpful to persons suffering from flatulence. Another variation: in the classical Shirsasana position open your knees and bend them backwards without pulling the muscles of the spinal area. Vatayasana or Pavanamuktasana is a particularly good posture for the practice of Asvini Mudra. Pavanamuktasana means 'the pose which releases the winds'. Lying on your back, bend both knees, placing your arms around them to bring them towards the chest. The thighs compress the abdomen and its contents. Practise Asvini Mudra in this position. If the intestines contain gas you can be sure of the result! Pavanamuktasana is no more than the final pose of Vatayasana.

Breathing
Asvini Mudra should preferably be synchronised with breathing. As we know, it can easily be combined with one of the main pranayama exercises with breath retention[*].

Asvini Mudra can also be performed as follows: (1) Inhalation (Puraka) - relaxed sphincter; (2) Kumbhaka (retention with full lungs) – dilate the sphincter; (3) Exhalation (Rechaka) – relaxed sphincter; (4) Kumbhaka (retention with empty lungs) – contraction of the sphincter. Practise this series for ten respirations. After a rest, start the same cycle again in reverse during breath retentions: Kumbhaka with full lungs – contract the sphincter; Kumbhaka with empty lungs – dilate the sphincter.

Hygienic effects
Asvini Mudra is the ideal exercise for strengthening the pelvic floor. By developing the muscles of the pelvic area and controlling them, the sagging of the rectum, of the uterus, of the vagina and of the bladder can be avoided. The alternate contraction and dilation of the sphincter itself prevents unpleasant haemorrhoids, since the veins of the anus are toned up and decongested.

This exercise is particularly important for expectant mothers because it affects the whole genital system. Deliveries are greatly helped if the pelvic floor is both strong and supple. Childbirth would be less painful if young women practised Asvini Mudra regularly. It is a very useful adjunct to the usual techniques for painless childbirth. The effect of Asvini Mudra (and of Mula Bandha) on the pelvic part of the parasympathetic nervous system is such that it efficiently combats constipation, their influence not being restricted to the autonomous nervous system which regulates the evacuation movements of the colon and of the rectum (peristalsis of the terminal part of the digestive tract), but extending to the muscles which co-operate inevacuating the faeces.

---

[*] See Section 21, pp. 128-132

Whatever philosophical or other considerations may be connected with the 'species' or the 'individual' poles, the purely physiological benefits derived from Mula Bandha can be explained anatomically and they are sufficient to justify its practice in pranayama.

The nervous control of our bodies receives orders on the one hand from the conscious and voluntary nervous system, and on the other hand from the autonomous nervous system which slows down or accelerates the functioning of the viscera. The latter, called autonomous because it was thought to be completely independent of the voluntary nervous system, is subdivided into: (1) *the sympathetic nerve* which runs along the spine from the dorsal vertebrae down to the first two lumbar vertebrae, innervates the heart and accelerates its beats, also affecting the digestive tract and its glands; (2) *the parasympathetic nerve* or vagus, which starts from the medulla oblongata at the base of the brain and also innervates most of these organs. The sympathetic and parasympathetic nerves are antagonistic. The latter retard the heartbeats and make them strong and slow. Thus, the visceral organism reacts and adapts itself to circumstances with infinite sensitivity, using either the brake or the accelerator. But the description is incomplete; reference to the pelvic parasympathetic nerve has been omitted.

Importance of the pelvic parasympathetic nerve
We might compare the human being to a plant which has its roots in the pelvis or, more precisely, in the sacrum, from which its long and flexible stem, the spine, rises. At the top, like a flower, is the brain, illuminated by the individual conscience. Mula Bandha is the contraction of the roots, of the base.

The sacrum constitutes the base of the whole skeleton. It is also, as we have seen, the seat of the 'species' pole, whereas the 'individual' pole is at the opposite end in the skull. The sacrum is much more than 'a large triangular bone'. It is composed of five sacral vertebrae fused together, which provide a passage for the sacral nerves whose importance cannot be overestimated. The nerve fibres which emerge join together like electric wires to form a larger 'cable' (the pelvic nerve) which goes through a transformer (the pelvic plexus) from which some nervous current is sent to all pelvic organs through conducting wires (the nerves). Some of these wires connect the descending colon, the rectum, the anus and the bladder (Apana). Other wires (vaso-dilating fibres) go to these organs and to the penis (the clitoris and the vulva in women) and to the muscles of the external genital organs. Therefore, the pelvic parasympathetic nerve controls certain strategic functions. If you carefully examine the diagram, you will be struck by the importance of the pelvic sympathetic nerve, and you will understand much better what happens in pranayama. During breath retention, the parasympathetic nerve is excited at its point of origin, in the bulb, at the base of the brain. We have studied the repercussions when describing Kumbhaka, the diving reflex, etc. That excitation gradually spreads to the whole parasympathetic system and increases the constructive (anabolic) functions of the body. However, the sacral and pelvic parts of the parasympathetic system escape this stimulation almost entirely, which is precisely what must be avoided. The whole system must be stimulated since a stimulation limited to its point of origin at the base of the brain might cause imbalance.

How can we extend the stimulation to the sacral and pelvic parts of the parasympathetic system? Through the practice of Asvini Mudra and Mula Bandha, which complement each other. Both affect the same parts of the body and have fairly similar pranic repercussions. What applies to one, from the viewpoint of the nervous mechanisms for instance, can be extended to the other. Both have an effect on the basic chakra, Mula-dhara, which will be studied with more detail later.

Since we are on the subject of anatomy, let us quote a paragraph from a book by a Dutch physician, Dr Rama Polderman, a yoga therapist:[*]

'Before winding up this lesson in anatomy we must turn our attention to the coccygean gland of Luschka, whose physiology and practical role are very little known. It is an irregular mass of cells situated at the tip of the coccyx. It is the size of a pea, oval-shaped. It is irrigated by capillaries and has autonomous nervous fibres. That gland resembles the carotid body placed in the neck close to the carotid artery, which influences blood pressure, breathing and sleep. The nerve which com-

---

[*] *Doe zelf de volgende stap in yoga*, p. 59

mands the carotid body is called Vijnanadi in yoga language.* The coccygean body performs a similar function. During Mula Bandha practice its nerve endings are stimulated. The coccygean body is linked. directly to the asymmetric ganglion – an autonomous nervous centre – by its nerve fibres. Hitherto Western physiology has paid only limited attention to this minute but very important structure. The carotid sinus has been studied more deeply and its physiological significance has been amply demonstrated. The yogis have known the function and usefulness of these two bodies for centuries.'

Technique
Asvini Mudra is the obligatory preparation for Mula Bandha. In fact, in Asvini Mudra the contraction is followed by a dilation, while in Mula Bandha contraction of the anal sphincter is both more powerful and more prolonged, which presents an additional difficulty. In reality it is not a difficulty, but as the muscles which lift the anus and the anal sphincter are structures not systematically exercised their power of contraction will increase through regular and progressive practice. Before we get to precise, practical indications, let us keep in mind the essential elements of Mula Bandha:

1 simultaneous and continuous contraction of the internal and external anal sphincters;
2 contraction of the muscles lifting the anus;
3 contraction of the 'pelvic floor' (see Asvini Mudra);
4 contraction of the lower abdomen to push back the viscera towards the sacrum;
5 Kumbhaka, that is breath retention with full lungs. This element is not indispensable as Mula Bandha is often maintained for a very long time, spreading over several pranayama. If one of the first four elements is missing, the efficacy and accuracy of the exercise are reduced proportionately.

Mula Bandha gives perfect control over this vital part of the body so that it can be ordered at will. Control can become so complete that it is possible to draw up water through the anus, expel it and evacuate

---

*   We have mentioned the carotid sinuses when studying Jalandhara Bandha. We find that everthing is linked and that bandhas form a structured and interdependent whole.

the contents of the colon, thus affecting a thorough cleasing of the intestines (Basti). People who do not practise such cleansing do not realise that the anus, the rectum and the colon are never free of residual faeces, which, because they become the sources of many illnesses that weaken the body and poison our lives,* should be eliminated. At first, bandha will be maintained for a few seconds only, but with training this period can be lengthened. One must then relax the muscle completely, that is, undo the bandha. It must be practised regularly twice a day, in series of twenty contractions. Thus complete mastery over this part of the body can be acquired with ensuing excellent health.

The bandha must also be practised immediately after going to the lavatory so as to expel the last residue that would otherwise remain in the colon. This is how to proceed: after a deep inhalation, hold your breath and contract the anus. When you cannot hold the air any longer, exhale and relax the sphincter. Repeat twenty times, as indicated above.

Mula Bandha may also be performed with the help of a chair. Sit astride a chair facing the back with your chest as close as possible to it, with your legs at the sides and your hands on the back. This must be done on an empty stomach. Perform the contractions as indicated above. To make sure you have gained control over the sphincter, try this very simple test: while you are inhaling, contract the sphincter and perform Mula Bandha, and maintain the contraction as long as you are holding your breath; when you exhale, try not to relax the muscles; maintain the bandha; if the sphincter is not completely under control, the bandha will tend to slacken by itself.

When performing Mula Bandha and Asvini Mudra, the student must contract both the sphincters which close the anus. There is the external anal sphincter which closes the extremity of the digestive tract, but it is essential to keep in mind that the anus has a second muscular ring, the internal sphincter situated two or three centimetres higher in the rectum. *Both sphincters must be contracted.* It is quite easy to be made aware of the two sphincters: focus your attention on the anus and contract it, then concentrate on a point slightly above this sphincter and contract it, and at that instant you will perceive an intense contraction of the whole anal area and of the perineum. Only then is Mula Bandha correct, though the books which mention

* Perfect cleanliness of the whole digestive tract is ensured by Shank Prakshalana, one of the rejuvenating methods described on p. 31 of *Je perfectionne mon Yoga.*

this detail are rare, if any. The contraction of the second sphincter is most important because the nerve endings which affect the colon, the abdominal wall and the diaphragm, in short all the organs which play a part when the faeces are evacuated, are situated just above this muscular ring. The efficiency of Mula Bandha depends on the simultaneous contraction of the two sphincters.

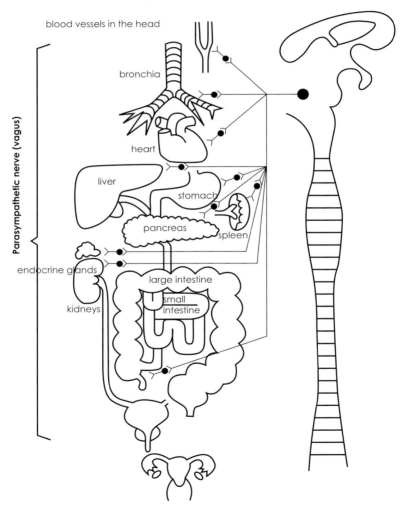

blood vessels in the head

bronchia

heart

liver

stomach

pancreas

spleen

endocrine glands

large intestine

small intestine

kidneys

Parasympathetic nerve (vagus)

3 6 | B a n d h a   T r a y a

Bandha Traya means 'the three bandhas'. In this exercise they are performed simultaneously, with maximum benefits. Bandha Traya is usually performed with empty lungs. The three bandhas combine in this order: Mula Bandha, Uddiyana Bandha, Jalandhara Bandha.

Uddiyanu Bandha
Uddiyana Bandha has been fully described in *Yoga Self-Taught*. Uddiyana is the Sanskrit expression 'to fly away'. During its practise one has the feeling that the stomach rises, literally 'flies away'upward. This bandha, like Mula Bandha, must be practised on an empty stomach and the most propitious time is after the morning asana session. Lean slightly forward, place your hands on your thighs, above the knees or close to the groin, and empty your lungs completely (the weight of the torso must rest on the arms). Then raise the diaphragm by false inhalation; the intestines are forced back towards the spine as the abdomen retracts. Hold it for a few seconds, then release the bandha and inhale again. This bandha is very important for the digestive tract; in a way, Mula Bandha and Uddiyana Bandha complete each other, since the organs concerned are closely related and perfectly synchronised. We should practise these bandhas together. After learning and mastering them separately they should be combined as a single exercise.

The best results are obtained by combining the three bandhas, that is by adding Jalandhara Bandha, the jugular contraction practised with empty lungs. It is possible for novices to start their training with full lungs because it is easier. When the lungs are filled with air, the ribs are lifted (which causes the thorax to expand), the neck is lowered until the chin exerts pressure on the body. To practise these bandhas, it is desirable to choose a quiet place where you will not be disturbed and where you will be alone, for concentration plays an essential part. When you practise the bandhas separately you must always concentrate on the muscles you are contracting whereas, if the three bandhas are combined, you must first concentrate on Mula Bandha, then on Uddiyana Bandha which is next, and finally on Jalandhara Bandha. Remain concentrated on the three bandhas. When they are released (in reverse order: first Jalandhara, then Uddiyana, finally Mula Bandha) concentrate on each bandha as it relaxes.

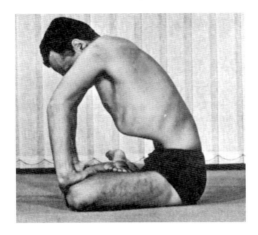

In Bandha Traya which combines Jalandhara, Mula and Uddiyana, the chin is slightly low-ered because of the particular curve of the back, shown in profile on the photograph

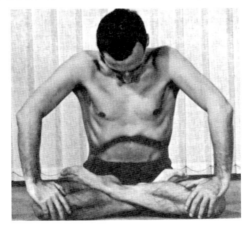

In this photograph the oblique abdominal muscles protrude.

In order to grasp the deep meaning of pranayama and its dimensions, which extend beyond the purely physiological framework, certain fundamental concepts of Indian thought must be assimilated. I should reassure Western readers that there is nothing here, however, that might offend their philosophical or religious beliefs. Also, I apologise for using a Sanskrit vocabulary, for there are words that have no exact equivalent in Western languages, even though they have the same Sanskrit origin.

The Indian concept of the structure of a human being is very elaborate, but we shall try to be as 'panoramic'as possible, that is to say, to bring out the main points and to leave the details to specialists. For thousands of years the wise men and thinkers of India have asked themselves the two questions 'Who am I?' and 'What am I?' For lack of a revealed truth, such as the Gospels and the Old Testament, they looked for the answer within themselves, through introspection and observation. Gradually penetrating deeper and deeper through the layers of body and psyche, they approached the inner self. They dissected and indentified the various components of their beings and their age-old empiricism is invaluable, not only from a theoretical viewpoint but also for practical purposes. We shall not attempt to describe, even sketchily, the slow process which led to the elaboration of this psycho-physiological system; we prefer to start directly with the large themes.

According to Indian thinkers and rishis the human being is composed of stratifications ranging from the most spiritual state of being to its most dense manifestation, the visible body. Each stratification is called a 'kosha', a word which we might be tempted to translate as a layer, but this might imply a separation of the various components, an idea alien to Indian thinking, which regards the human being as an indivisible whole. As human beings we possess a visible material body composed of identifiable atoms and molecules; but, as opposed to the molecules and atoms of the non-organic universe, these material particles are structured into a bodily form itself animated by a mysterious vital energy. We perceive, we think, we love, we suffer, we walk, we eat, but above all we change. Let us repeat once more that we are never twice exactly identical to ourselves, either from the viewpoint of material composition or mentally. And the whole structure says 'me–I'

Let us see how the Indians understand this biophysical complex. True, we are dealing with an individual, with a life centre separated, at least apparently, from the other individuals who may or may not be the same species. But where is the source? For Indian thinkers the densest layers originate from the most spiritual stratifications, these being causal in their relationship to the others. In a way the Indian approach runs counter to that of Western science: it looks through the other end of the telescope. For Western science consciousness is undoubtedly sited in the brain and is considered a side-product of cortical activity. For yogis and Indian thinkers, on the contrary, the brain is but the instrument of the mind, where it is situated rather than vice versa. Mind manufactures the brain and uses it, and the brain is in the mind. Absurd? Paradoxical? But before we reach a verdict we must bear in mind that a primitive person, listening to a radio set for the first time, would undoubtedly believe that the person who is talking is inside the set; but for us the radio set is tuned to receive waves and is merely the instrument for the manifestation of sound waves. Indian thinkers believe our causal layer, our deepest kosha, to be the source of all others, to be Anandamaya Kosha.

Anandamaya Kosha
The source of all other koshas, Anandamaya Kosha is characterised by the absolute felicity (ananda) which surrounds Jivatman with a halo. Jivatman is composed of *Jiva*, Sanskrit for 'man', and *atman* corresponding to the concept of 'soul'; thus Jivatman is the soul of man, our very essence. It is the Self, with a capital S, of the human being. Jivatman is the profound Spectator and the hidden architect of all the other stratifications. Its nature is the pure consciousness, a concept which escapes our Western thinking. Anandamaya Kosha is outside time and space. Jivatman is placed beyond chance events and pairs of opposites.

According to Indian thought man is not a body and a soul; he is a soul that built himself a body, a concept not opposed to Christian ideas. The only fundamental difference is that for Christian thought the soul has only one contact with matter, only one incarnation. For the Indian thinker the soul is caught up in a round of successive births and deaths, each time resuming contact with matter when its corporal instruments have disintegrated in death. The reader will object that this 'sole' difference is sizeable. Agreed; yet if we keep to the structure of a well-defined individual, to an incarnation, there is no great difference from a structural viewpoint. Therefore we can forget this dfference of concepts. It is from this dynamic centre that the successive layers will materialise. This causal layer is not physically observable and therefore will never be an object for scientific study. Psychology does not mention it.

Vijnanamaya Kosha

In its dynamic process of materialisation, Jivatman, or the soul, at first creates an individual centre for itself and undergoes a first densification: Vijnanamaya Kosha. This kosha is structured around the concept of Ahamkara, which means the sense of ego, or the self (with a small s) of modern psychology. It is this mysterious faculty which makes me conscious of the fact that I am an individual, a centre of consciousness separate from others. It is the principle of individualisation. Me-I is the reference centre to which all life experiences are related, just as the spokes of a wheel are related to the axle. When I was born, I was quite different physically and mentally from what I am now. In a few years, I shall be different again. And yet, I shall be present. This profound sense of individualisation, this permanent reference centre, is the pivot around which Vijnanamaya Kosha is organised (approximate translation: intellect, reason). 'I think, therefore I am' has its place in Vijnanamaya Kosha. It is at the same level that conscience is found. By conscience we mean the sense of what is right and wrong and not the conscious part of our mental activity. Reason (Buddhi) is also situated there.

Manomaya Kosha

Vijnanamaya Kosha and Manomaya Kosha overlap and interpenetrate. Manomaya Kosha is the whole psychic activity except that which is included in the concept of Vijnanamaya Kosha. It contains all our psychic instruments for the perception of the outside world. It constitutes our mind (the one studied by modern psychology) which evolves parallel with the body. It also includes our instincts, inherited from our ancestors, as well as all individual traits acquired since our birth. It comprises our complexes, our conscious sensations and our individual subconscious. This is the layer psychoanalysts try to reach. It also includes the contents of our memory accumulated since we were born. When I dream I am conscious and my memory functions, since

I can recall the contents of my dreams when I wake up. I can have feelings when I dream, I can be frightened or gay, depending on the nature of the dream. Everything that participates in the dream - my unconscious, my ability to create mental pictures, everything that conditions the contents of my dreams (my unconscious impulses, my memories, my inhibited desires, etc.) – is part of Manomaya Kosha. When I dream, my intellect does not function, nor does my reason. I may dream that I am flying like a bird without being surprised because my reason and my intellect (Vijnanamaya Kosha) do not work during dreams. Manomaya Kosha also comprises my psychic instruments of action. I want to express myself, to be active in the outside world. Behind my moving body there is the animator, a mind with its deep motivations.

To make things easier, Vijnanamaya Kosha and Manomaya Kosha may be considered as the psychic layer. They constitute what the occultists call the astral body, an ambiguous expression we prefer not to use.

Whereas the causal kosha (Anandamaya Kosha) is situated outside time and space (the soul is immortal), the psychic body has but one dimension. It is non-spatial but it is temporal. While I am sleeping, my dream does not take up x cubic metres. Still, dreams occupy time since it is possible to tell, within seconds, from an encephalogram, at what time the dream started and when it ended. Incidentally, the time of dreams is quite different from the time on the clock. A dream which actually lasts a short time on the clock may give the impression that it had lasted for several hours! Similarly, our feelings have no volume, no weight. How many ounces does a fit of anger weigh? The question is absurd of course. It is precisely because our minds are dimensionless that they can bring together, into one global perception, sensations from various parts of the cerebral outer layer, corresponding to the perception centres of the cortex.

Pranamaya Kosha and Annamaya Kosha
Let us consider making a movement. Immediately skeleton, muscles and tendons are put into action. All of which is very natural, no doubt, but on reflection so mysterious! How can the intangible thought set these material particles in motion? This is what we are going to demonstrate. We shall first of all examine the densest layer, the corporal layer, Annamaya Kosha.

We know by analysis, that the human body is composed approximately of 65 per cent oxygen, 18 per cent carbon, 10 per cent hydrogen, 3 per cent nitrogen, 2 per cent calcium, 1 per cent phosphorous, totalling 99 per cent. The remaining 1 per cent represents twenty-three other elements ranging from iron to titanium and including cobalt, nickel and molybdenum. Those are the material components of our body. Where do they come from? From our food, naturally, if we understand it in the sense of solid, liquid or gaseous nourishment. By definition, these material elements are inert. They are grouped and put into action by forces called pranas. Pranamaya Kosha (please note it is not pranayama) is our spiritual yet material pranic body. All the electrical, magnetic or other forces which are at work in our bodies give it the appearance of life. Some electric currents run through the material layer (Annamaya Kosha) along lines of force and material conductors.

Because it is the densest layer, Annamaya Kosha is often scorned: this is an error the Western world has been committing for centuries. And yet the molecular body, Annamaya Kosha, is the one kosha where all other koshas come together. It is the sacred stage on which the cosmic drama of human life unfolds. Without it, human manifestation on the terrestrial level would be impossible. It conditions the aspect and perfection of man's manifestation in the totality. Annamaya Kosha is permeated and impregnated by mind (of which it is the expression). The aim of yoga is to make it as perfect as possible and to spiritualise it, but these two layers are in themselves inert. They are quadridimensional. They exist in time and space and dissolve entirely with death, in order to return at once to the physical world. The true motive power behind the movements of Annamaya Kosha (the layer formed by food) and Pranamaya (the energising layer) is mind (Manomaya and Vijnanamaya Koshas). The places where psychic forces act upon the inferior layers and come into contact with them are the 'chakras'.

Chakras

The comparison – already made – with a radio set enables us to grasp by analogy a very important notion in matters of pranayama: the transposition of an activity taking place at a particular level to another level. Radio (or television) waves correspond to a certain activation of the electromagnetic field. By acting upon a particular structure (the radio set) by means of another type of energy (the electric current in the set), the vibration of the electromagnetic field comes out in the form of gross vibrations of the air around us, vibrations which can be perceived by the human ear. And yet these various activities are superimposed in space: the inaudible radio waves take up the whole volume of the room where I am listening to them as sound waves. The vibration of the electromagnetic field has become an air vibration without ceasing to be a vibration of the electromagnetic field. Both vibrations are superimposed in space. Similarly, psychic dynamism manifests itself (movements of the body) through the chakras and the pranic body.

The process is reversible. An air vibration (the voice of a speaker), intercepted by a microphone and transformed by the transmitter, is changed into radio waves. The various koshas represent just as many existence levels of the human being, they intermingle, they are superimposed and act upon one another without becoming mixed. This is an example of the transformation of psychic energy into physical movement.

One man insults another. Anger (one dimension only, time) rises in the mind of the offended party. It affects certain centres of nervous and cerebral energy (chakras) which start a whole chain of pranic reactions: his face becomes red with anger because of the uprush of blood; he clenches his fists. Should anger increase in intensity, an exchange of blows might ensue: the nadis have ordered the movements of molecules and atoms in the muscles of the offender.

A yogi is one who is capable of consciously passing from one level to another, or rather of controlling with his will and his consciousness all these processes and of increasing or decreasing their intensity as he wishes. This is called mastery of the body and the spirit and is the very essence of yoga. A yogi may also slow down activity at all levels (koshas) and retire within himself in Anandamaya Kosha, 'the profound spectator', or rather he lets 'the profound spectator' isolate himself temporarily from anything which is not his essence. He thus experiences absolute felicity (Ananda). It is the supreme experience: the Samadhi. At that moment the 'spectator' comes into contact with the entire cosmos without passing through the intermediary of his senses. Some secrets which may afterwards modify the functioning of materialisation koshas (that is all the other koshas) may then be revealed to him. That is why the yoga tradition proclaims that it is an ordinary man who goes into Samadhi and a sage who comes out of it. The modification of materialisation koshas is in fact the sign of true

Samadhi: a simple slowing down (without modification) of the koshas, without supreme experience, may in all good faith be considered as Samadhi.

It might be advisable to summarise and quickly reconstruct the whole, but this time starting from the densest elements. Composed of the material elements produced by food, Annamaya Kosha is penetrated, animated and controlled by Pranamaya Kosha (the whole of the pranic forces) travelling along the hundreds of thousands of nadis. Pranamaya Kosha is, in turn, governed and penetrated by Manomaya Kosha and Vijnanamaya Kosha (mental body) which give to it conscious and unconscious thought and the sense of the 'me'. My arm rises because pranic energy makes it rise under the influence of a thought. Whatever the motivation that makes me raise my arm, it belongs to the psychic universe.

This is where the chakras come in. Together with the nadis they are one of the most prolific subjects of yoga literature, though their nature is not well defined. The chakras are the contact points where the mental body integrates with the energising body (Pranamaya Kosha). Chakras are spiritual energy centres where psychic dynamism comes into contact with the inert elements (the dense body and the pranic body) and controls them, and where psychic forces change their manifestation level.

In order to clarify our thinking we shall resume our analogy of the radio set. The electromagnetic field of radio waves vibrates at a given frequency but is inaudible to the human ear; to materialise them, we need an intermediary, the radio set. Although the entire set is in contact with the radio waves which surround it, the aerial constitutes a particular point where the waves penetrate the set. This particular contact point acts like a chakra in the radio set: from this chakra the waves are carried along the circuits (nadis) by the energy of the radio set (prana) which comes from the batteries or the electricity supply. Finally, the loudspeaker manifests the waves which thus passed from the 'spiritual' to the 'gross' level.

It is no different for a human being. The mental body is the radio wave, the chakras are the points where mental energy penetrates the pranic body and forms a vortex (*chakra*: wheel, vortex in Sanskrit). The mental layers meet and control the energising and dense layers at the chakras, which are both centres of energy and of consciousness. In an average man, chakras and nadis function automatically without the intervention of the conscious and voluntary self. In a yogi, not only does consciousness penetrate these vortexes but it is capable of increasing the mental energy pressure wherever it wishes, on the material as well as on the spiritual level. That is why a true yogi is an extra-ordinary being in the strictest sense. The chakras have to be in contact with the nadis. They are like transformer stations in an electricity supply system.

Psychic chakras live only as long as we do, although they have material, physical supports. They may be studied and described either as anatomic structures or as perception centres, depending on whether they are perceived in the psychic or in the anatomic layer. An interesting comparison could be made between acupuncture and the chakras but unfortunately it is not possible for us to do so. We have seen that some nadis correspond to the meridians of acupuncture. The Chinese points or centres, where the gold or silver needles are applied by the acupuncturist to act on the lines of force carried by the meridians, are chakras. Consequently there are thousands of chakras in the human body. As with the nadis, although it is not absolutely necessary to launch into a complex study, it is essential to know the main chakras. From here we realise the vast scope of pranayama, of the dynamics of breathing.

The various pranayama exercises modify the conditions of absorption of prana, of circulation along the nadis, of accumulation and distribution through the chakras, but the main dynamic element is the mind. Carried out without concentration, pranayama exercises are only hygienic respiratory activities, but with the help of concentration they permit full manifestation of the resources of our psychic dynamism on a terrestrial level. The pranic body (Pranamaya Kosha) is therefore a special stratification in our human structure: that is why yoga is unthinkable without pranayama. Control of the superior layers is impossible without the integration and conscious control of the so-called inferior layers. But we must not believe that those layers are separate like the layers of an onion; they interpenetrate and their action is reversible, either from the mind to the dense outer world or from the dense outer world to the psychic universe. Thus the 'I' passes from one level to another. The 'profound spectator' is like a grain of sand in the oyster; it is the hidden and forgotten cause of the pearl. Thus Jivatman creates tools for itself and hides in them. The soul creates a body and animates it. What transcends time and space and therefore is immortal is man, the 'profound spectator'. All other things are his tools, his 'body' (psychic, mental, pranic and dense). Thus, going down from one level to another, the 'spectator' comes into contact with denser and denser layers without itself becoming temporal or spatial. The radio waves continue to affect the whole electromagnetic field, even when they come into contact with a receiving set which materialises them. They reach the level of manifestation without leaving the level of the electromagnetic waves, themselves inaudible to the human ear.

Pranayama could be described as the psycho-physiological process of the activation of the various chakras, accompanied by the awakening of the consciousness of these energy centres.

Causal layer

Anandamaya Kosha
Causal stratification. Its nature is *joy* and pure *felicity*, beyond qualities. Its centre is Jivatman (the soul of man), the profound architect-spectator.

Mental or spiritual body

Vijnanamaya Kosha
Seat of the Ego (Ahamkara, the principle of individualisation in man). Its instruments are: intellect and Buddhi (reason, discernment). This stratification can act on Manomaya Kosha and counterbalance for example the unconscious impulses, and can inhibit or control the instincts. It is the permanent reference centre. When a human being says 'I think that I think', that is a reflective action due to Vijnana Maya Kosha.

Manomaya Kosha
This is mind in general, or the mechanisms of the wakeful consciousness, the unconscious with its impulses and its instincts, its complexes, studied by Western psychology. It comprises perception and action instruments. It also comprises individual memory and memory inherited from our ancestors. Manomaya Kosha commands the movements of the body. Its psychic dynamism acts on pranic stratification through the chakras, which are transformation centres for mental energy.

Gross or dense body

Pranamaya Kosha
Is composed of all the forces at work in the human body. With the action impulses coming from Manomaya Kosha, it sets the dense elements of the body in motion. Forces move along the nadis. That energising layer is inert and insensitive. It is the Manomaya Kosha's instrument of action.

Annamaya Kosha
The densest stratification of the human being. Is composed of chemical elements (atoms, molecules) coming from food (solid food, drinks, oxygen in the air). Inert and dense, it is the instrument of action and manifestation of the superior stratifications.

Correlation with the Christian doctrine: Anandamaya Kosha corresponds to the soul. The other stratifications are the spiritual and dense aspects of the body.

The superior koshas interpenetrate and comprise the inferior layers. Annamaya Kosha and Pranamaya Kosha have four dimensions (three space dimensions + time).

Manomaya Kosha and Vijnanamaya Kosha exist only in time.

Ananda Maya Kosha is beyond time and space.

By controlling the incoming current and the switches on the instrument panel of a computer I control the entire circulation and utilisation of electrical energy within the apparatus and I regulate its work. Similarly, by having in check a limited number of key chakras we control the whole of the dense and pranic bodies.

Some chakras are connected with the 'species' pole in the pelvis, others with the 'individual' pole in the brain. The two poles are linked by the main prana conductors, the nadis, Pingala, Ida, and Sushumna. Other chakras are placed along their course, each one controlling a portion of the total pranic circuit.

The chakra we are going to study first is more particularly linked to the species pole which is the root - or Muladhara Chakra (*Mula* = root; *Adhara* = support.) Therefore, Muladhara Chakra is the chakra which supports the root of a human being considered as a whole, and not only as a dense body. This energy centre is especially privileged since it is situated at the origin of the three principal nadis, and is the seat of Kundalini, the latent energy of the species within each living being. It is also one of the main organs of Apana.

We have already seen that the balance between Prana Vayu and Apana Vayu is essential for the pranic equilibrium of the body, spiritual and physical. Apana Vayu can be controlled most efficiently at Muladhara Chakra, that it, at the anus. Therefore, Muladhara Chakra represents the strategic crossroads in the pranic structure and in the framework of the chakras.

Is it not surprising that Kundalini should have chosen the least noble part of the body as its seat? The answer to this question will also settle another question which is often discussed in works dealing with pranayama, as to whether the chakras are situated inside or outside the spine? Actually Kundalini does not reside in the anus but in the nervous centres which command the rectum, the anus, the bladder and the genital organs. Remember the pelvic parasympathetic system mentioned in our study on Asvini Mudra. It is impossible to command the pelvic parasympathetic system directly, but the will can act on its extremity, the anal sphincter, and from there on the nervous centre itself (pelvic plexus) and on the nervous centres of the sacral marrow. The centre of the sexual reflex is found in the spinal marrow, enclosed in the sacrum. By working on the terminal pole – the anus and the perineum – a yogi indirectly works on the nervous control centre, the sacral plexus which is the true seat of Kundalini, or rather the contact point between Kundalini (spiritual and cosmic energy of the species) and the nervous centres of the individual in the sacrum. It is impossible for a neophyte or an uninitiated person to be conscious of the plexus itself. Through exercises which activate this chakra via the most remote extremities and with the help of special Kriya Yoga techniques, a yogi can awaken this chakra; he succeeds in perceiving and becoming conscious of the centre itself (the nervous plexus). This consciousness creates impressions appearing as colours which must be unreal, since they do not result from external luminous stimulations. A vibration can be perceived too. That is why yogis have described the colours of this chakra and have transposed the vibrations they perceived into syllables. The visual impressions are unstable and seem to turn and whirl around. Hence the use of the term 'chakra', meaning also a wheel or a vortex. Chakras are sometimes symbolised by a lotus because those unreal colours evoke flowers. For yogis, particularly tantric yogis, a human being (microcosm) reflects the macrocosm (universe). Individual energy is a microcosmic manifestation of a macrocosmic energy which is symbolically represented as a goddess. Each chakra is the seat of a specialised form of energy both psychic (in its Manomaya Kosha aspect) and energising (Pranamaya Kosha); this energy has been symbolised and personified by yoga adepts as a goddess. As a consequence there are various pictures representing the chakras, but they are, needless to say, purely subjective and influenced by the religious and philosophical backgrounds of those who have experienced them. It would be a mistake to take these portrayals literally and transpose them into the Western world along the lines in which they are portrayed in India and have been published by Arthur Avalon.

In our study of chakras we shall describe the anatomical connection (whenever possible and when authors agree), the psychic counterpart and, in the case of Muladhara Chakra, the cosmic counterpart.

At the base of the sacrum there is, besides the sacral plexus mentioned above, an important nerve centre at the junction with the coccyx. A number of nerve endings, motor and receptor, intermingle there. Through the practice of appropriate exercises and starting from the nerve endings (motor and receptor) of the anal sphincter, the student cannot fail to reach the real command centre, wherever it may be. The contraction of the anal sphincter and of the perineum also works on the sexual organs of men and women alike and consequently on the centres which command reflex sexual activity in the spinal marrow. That is why in pictures of the root chakra we find the lingam (male organ) symbolising the male creative aspect of the cosmos, itself represented by Shiva, only the symbol of a cosmic force and not a god in the Western sense. The lingam is placed in a triangle pointing downwards. The triangle represents yoni – the female sex organ – and through it the universal cosmic female aspect. It also represents nature, the creative Shakti. The female and male cosmic aspects meet in the basic chakra. In India, everyone knows that an inverted triangle symbolises yoni. As India was evolving toward some kind of continence (not to be confused with chastity for they are two quite different things) some masters cheated a bit. Instead of representing Muladhara Chakra according to tradition – an inverted triangle with the lingam and the snake – they forgot about the lingam and had the triangle pointed upwards! One of these masters was Swami Sivananda, to my knowledge the first to modify the traditional image. Later others (mostly Western) copied this revised and corrected drawing. But there was a reason for the revision: Swami Sivananda, as a monk in charge of an ashram where continence was compulsory, probably loathed the traditional image. There was in India, especially among Dravidians (the only truly indigenous and original group) a shaktic cult which gave birth to tantrism. It includes certain sexual practices and rituals and led to excesses which started a reaction and brought discredit on tantrism. This was justified so far as the excesses were concerned, yet extremely unjust otherwise, according to Arnaud Desjardins, because trantrism represents, in our age of Kali, the most authentic way of returning to the cosmic source of our being. However, it is not necessary to be interested in tantrism in order to work on Muladhara Chakra.

Some masters (only modern ones and usually monks) warned disciples against the use of this chakra. With all respect, they are probably wrong. If the individual pole alone is activated an imbalance ensues and man is cut off from his very source, from roots which go deep into the species and its creative, evolutionary dynamism. For Kundalini also represents the evolutionary force which guides the modifications of all the species. Kundalini contains all present and future potentialities for the evolution of human beings. It would be just as wrong to activate the root chakra only. Electric current comes from a difference of potential between two poles. So it is for human beings too.

Summary
Muladhara Chakra, the root chakra, is the point of contact of the species pole in human beings, the point of departure of the three main nadis (Ida, Pingala and Sushumna) and one of the principal organs active in Apana-Vayu, the eliminating activity of the body which must be balanced with Prama-Vayu, the entry of prana into human beings in all its forms. Practical applications are found in Asvini Mudra and Mula Bandha, as well as in the Kriyas which allow the activation of this chakra.

Now, after Muladhara Chakra, we shall study its opposite pole, Sahasrara Chakra, the chakra of the individual pole, situated in the brain. If it is possible, from descriptions in ancient treatises linked with our own anatomical knowledge, to localise the root chakra and a few others with some degree of precision, the same may not be said of Sahasrara; we only know that it is situated in the brain. However, as a point of contact and of dynamic exchange between Manomaya Kosha and the command centre of the individual pole, it is possible to become aware of it without too much difficulty; that is more important than finding its actual anatomical site, which has purely academic interest.

Between root chakra and Sahasrara Chakra the liaison circuit is composed of Ida, Pingala and Sushumna. The other chakras are spaced along this axis like towns along a motorway. Continuous exchanges of pranic energy take place along it. By controlling these two opposite chakras, a yogi gains mastery over all the other chakras and their activation, and indirectly over the whole organism.

Awareness of Sahasrara Chakra

This is the technique designed to give you an awareness of Sahasrara Chakra. Sitting in a pranayama asana with straight spine, start breathing calmly. When breathing is even and peaceful, direct your inner gaze into the cranium. Concentrate your thought on a point within the head, half-way along an imaginary line between the temples. With a little practice and patience and by focusing all your attention on that area, you will perceive some pulsations. With prolonged practice, some subtle sounds and luminous sensations can be experienced but that is neither indispensable nor important. It is simply a possibility. Should you fail to sense the pulsations in your head, you can practise as follows: first place the fingertips on the temples in order to become aware of the arteries. Concentrate on this spot and try to feel the beats as clearly as possible. Then move your fingers away and practise perceiving the throbbing of the arteries in the temples without finger contact. It is not very difficult. When this has been achieved and concentration on this spot is no longer a problem, imagine that the beats spread gradually inside your head until the two pulsations meet half-way between the temples. That is the quickest and easiest way of being able to perceive the beats in that area. Pulsations are sometimes felt at the top of the cranium, which is quite normal.

Sahasrara Chakra occupies the whole encephalon; but it is not the brain, which is only its instrument, its physical counterpart. Because luminous impressions are readily perceptible there it is represented as a luminous lotus with innumerable petals. The number of one thousand which is mentioned in the texts must not be taken literally; it means 'many' or 'innumerable' and we should not give it mathematical precision.

Sushumna
This is the main prana channel (nadi) and a lot of ink has been used on this subject. It is true that the tantrics place its origin in the heart, but yoga scriptures almost unanimously place its starting-point in Muladhara, from which Sushumna moves westward. According to the initiates' code, west means the posterior side of the body, explained by the fact that yogis always practise with their face turned towards the east; thus the side of the body lit by the rising sun is the 'east' side and the back becomes the 'west', and Paschima (west) in Paschimottanasana signifies stretching the west side, or backstretching.

To revert to Sushumna; leaving Muladhara it moves backward, that is to say towards the sacrum, then travels up the length of the spine. On emerging from the spine – in the cranium – Sushumna divides into two branches, one of them travelling towards the top of the head (Brahmarandra), where the hair forms a crown, the other rejoining Ajna Chakra (between the eyes). Sushumna may be partly identified with the spinal marrow but not exclusively, only for its course through the spine. Sushumna represents the flow of nervous energy passing from the anus to the sacrum, following the spinal marrow and prolonged towards the higher centres of the brain.

It is of relatively little practical importance to determine the exact course of Sushumna or to place the chakras with precision. The treatises also mention that Sushumna 'pierces' various chakras on its way, which implies that the latter are situated within the spine, whereas other descriptions place them outside. It is quite possible that the nervous centre in the spine is activated more particularly by a given chakra (the chakra being on the borderline between the anatomical and the psychic body. However, if we concentrate on a definite organ or area outside the spine, say on the heart beat, its repercussions are to be found along Sushumna. In other words, methods of chakra activation based on the exterior concept of Sushumna are perfectly acceptable and do not invalidate the hypothesis according to which the chakras are inside Sushumna.

The importance of Sushumna in yoga is considerable. In ordinary man pranic currents move mainly in Ida and Pingala, but a yogi seeks to attract Prana and Apana and make them move within Sushumna. To be conscious of the spine is essential and the practice of asanas with concentration on the unrolling of the vertebrae during the dynamic phases is an important factor. Here the emphasis on asanas as a preparation for pranayama appears once again.

The mental image is most important for guiding the energy along the spine. Yogis imagine Sushumna as a hollow tube inside the spine. On hearing the word 'imagine', the uninitiated conclude it is a question of autosuggestion purely and simply. In fact, if I imagine I am sending prana towards my hands, I actually send blood to them and they warm up. The mental image precedes and reinforces the physiological function. The importance given to Sushumna stems from the fact that it pierces the chakras, which neither Ida nor Pingala do. In ordinary man, not trained in yoga techniques, the chakras are independent centres, working automatically and unconsciously, sometimes in correlation with each other but always unknown to the person and therefore without his conscious control, just like the intestine. By guiding Apana and Prana into Sushumna, a yogi achieves conscious mastery over prana and the chakras; on the way he awakens some subtle psychic forces. Thus it is more with a view to activating mental and spiritual energies that these practices are followed.

Sushumna has another vital importance. When activated by a yogi, Sushumna synthesises the action of Ida and of Pingala and establishes a liaison between the centres of the species and individual poles. It is an excellent purifying agent, making possible the integration of all the main chakras at all levels. Kundalini also moves along Sushumna when it is awakened - an extremely rare occurrence. Therefore, safety will be found in the opening of Sushumna, an opening achieved through awareness, patient labour and perseverance. This may take years: let us have no illusions about it.

All attempts to identify chakras with precise organic structures, however attractive this may be, do not stand thorough examination and, what is more, do not agree with yogis' experiments or with the classical yoga texts. Identification with the plexuses appears to be the most plausible and the closest to yoga theory but there are great discrepancies which make it unacceptable in general. These attempts at identification originate from the assumption that chakras are organs whereas in fact they are energy centres (not only physical but psychic energy centres). Chakras are as much part of Manomaya Kosha – our unidimensional psychic structure – as of Pranamaya Kosha, the pranic body. Their activation takes place principally in the psyche, in the mind, which also explains *the importance of the role given* to mental work, to consciousness. We therefore include in the chakra concept: (1) a centre in the mental stratification (Manomaya Kosha); (2) its point of contact with Pranamaya Kosha; (3) its course in the nadis, especially Ida and Pingala, then in less important nadis which take it to its termination, which is (4) the organ or organs of resonance (the same chakra may have several organs of resonance).

Thus, Muladhara Chakra has its terminal point of resonance in the anus; its pranic course goes towards the sacrum. From there, it travels up toward the brain and the cerebral command centres. When a yogi performs Mula Bandha, he is conscious of his act: the contraction is wilful (therefore it has a counterpart in the brain and in the mind). The mere fact of thinking about Muladhara immediately establishes an energising circuit between the extremity to be activated (the anus) and the cerebral command centres. From a practical viewpoint, the exact course is not important. When we dial a telephone number and receive an answer at the other end, it is the connection that matters. Apart from the telephone company, no one worries about the real route of the conversation along the wires, or the power source, etc. Similarly, when practising chakra activation, the terminal pole and its conscious counterpart are essential and contact is automatically established as soon as we concentrate and project our willpower.

After studying the two polar chakras (Muladhara and Sahasrara) and outlining the importance of Sushumna – the great vital axis connecting these two poles – we can start on the other main chakras.

How many are there? Most books on yoga mention only six. Let us paya well deserved tribute to Sir John Woodroffe (Arthur Avalon) and his monumental work, *The Serpent Power*, which describes six of them (all authors have adopted his classification). There are actually hundreds, if not thousands of chakras, and to determine which are the most important ones is therefore a matter of personal evaluation.

The six chakras selected by Arthur Avalon certainly are the main ones but it is advisable to add two others, seldom described but important from a practical point of view, because they are included in the special kriyas which are meant to activate chakras. The two chakras we are adding to Avalon's six are Surya Chakra (the Solar Chakra)and Chandra Chakra (the Lunar Chakra).

Svadisthana Chakra

What is the etymology of this word? *Sva* means 'which is its own' (which belongs to oneself) and *Disthana* means 'its actual seat'. Whose seat? Kundalini's! Therefore the two chakras are inseparably linked and are very close to each other. By working on Muladhara Chakra, we work at the same time on Svadisthana since this chakra is situated immediately above Muladhara Chakra. According to yoga texts, it lies slightly above and in front of Muladhara. In accordance with more reliable sources available to us, we shall say it is placed at the root of the penis (lingam) for men, and for women in the uterus or at the root of the clitoris (the female homologue of the lingam).

Both Muladhara and Svadisthana Chakra are also dominated by Apana Vayu, the excretory energy. That is probably why some authors place them in the seminal vesicle. The organ corresponding to Svadisthana Chakra would then be placed in the lumbar area, the real command centre. The pelvic organs are governed by the pelvic parasympathetic nerve about which we have written at length, but also by the fibres originating in the lumbar marrow. During excretion (stool, urine, ejaculation) the pelvic parasympathetic nerve is active. Mula Bandha works exclusively on these reflex centres of the sacrum. When one refrains from moving the bowels, from urinating or ejaculating, the reflex centres of the lower dorsal lumbar marrow inhibit Apana Vayu. The nervous fibres which emerge from these centres join together at the lower mesenteric ganglion. Control of Muladhara and Svadisthana Chakra ensures control over excretory forces, sexual reflexes and Apana Vayu.

Manipura Chakra

In literal translation, 'The City of Jewels'! *Mani*: Jewel (remember the famous Buddhistic mantra *Om Mani Padme Hum*: O the jewel in the lotus). *Pura* means 'town, city'. The name indicates the importance of this chakra, sometimes called Nabhi Chakra, the chakra of the umbilicus, because yogis achieve mastery over it by concentrating on the umbilicus. Patanjali wrote in his aphorisms: *Nabhichakra Kayavyuha Jnanam*, meaning 'Continuous concentration on the navel provides knowledge of the entire body.'

Manipura Chakra is governed by Sarnana Vayu, the prana of food assimilation. The concentration activation of this chakra gives control over the whole assimilation of food. Therefore this chakra controls the stomach, the liver and the small intestine but stops at the colon. Wilhelm Reich wrote in *La Fonction de L'Orgasme* (L'Arche, Paris 1952, p. 232):

'There must be a vegetative centre where bioelectrical energy (prana) starts and returns. The abdominal cavity, the place attributed to emotions, contains generators of biological energy (chakras). These are large centres of the independent nervous system, particularly the solar plexus, the hypogastric plexus and the sacro-lumbar or pelvic plexus. A glance at the neuro-vegetative system shows that the vegetative ganglions are most dense in the abdominal and genital areas.'

Is the 'central vegetative centre' discovered by Reich any other than the Manipura Chakra of the yogis?

Some authors place Manipura Chakra in the solar plexus. Are they right or wrong? We know how risky it is to establish an identity between a definite chakra and a precise anatomical structure. Mastery over Manipura Chakra is achieved by concentrating on the navel area. In fact, when during pranayama exercises with prolonged breath retention (with full lungs) the student reaches the stage when it ceases to be comfortable, some reflex contractions occur in the abdominal wall and especially in the umbilical area, where vibrations are felt. If retention is carried still further, contraction and vibrations spread to Svadisthana and Muladhara Chakra. This is as far as a Western student may venture, provided he progresses slowly and practises both pranayama and asanas regularly; also provided that he is in perfect physical condition.

Suya Chakra and Chandra Chakra

Surya Chakra is the solar chakra (*Surya* means sun in Sanskrit). Less important than Manipura, whose action it completes, it is situated on the right, near the liver, slightly above the navel. Exactly like manipulation Chakra, Surya Chakra is the seat of Samana Vayu, the assimilating energy of the organism.

Chandra Chakra is its polar chakra since *Chandra* means moon in Sanskrit. In relation to the navel, it is symmetrical with Surya Chakra, therefore slightly to the left and above. Their balanced action, which is correlated with Manipura Chakra, is indispensable for the perfect functioning of Samana Vayu, the assimilatory energy.

Anahata Chakra

This is the heart chakra, whose activation is achieved through aware-ness and concentration on the heartbeats. The heart is considered the seat of' Jivatman', the individual soul. To point oneself out one directs the index finger towards the heart, not towards the brain. Yogis place the seat of the personality there but this assertion should not be taken literally. It is obviously not in the organ itself that our personality, our individual soul, is situated but it is the energy which causes the heart to beat which is directly linked to our individuality. It is probably because the heart immediately answers the emotions with a modification of its beats that we associate its action with the movements of the soul. It is therefore by meditating on 'that' which makes the heart beat rather than on the piece of flesh called heart that a yogi becomes conscious of his deep Self. Concentration on the 'mystic heart' has played a large part in the mystical techniques of the Christian Western world. Christ is pictured with a radiant heart. It is obvious that the Christian mystics did not have the physical heart in view but its psychic counterpart.

Vishuddha Chakra

This chakra's resonance centre is in the throat and more precisely in the pharynx and the vocal cords. Its deeper centre lies in the cervical spine and it is activated by becoming conscious of that area. It controls Udana Vayu, that is to say all aspects of psychophysical energy which lead to vocal expression. When man expresses his thoughts, Udana Vayu is working. We talk, thanks to Udana Vayu, whose area is not just limited to the vocal cords but extends to the whole zone including the throat and the mouth as well as the face. Every facial expression depends on Udana Vayu. Breathing in Ujjayi is an effective means of controlling this chakra.

Ajna Chakra

This lies between the eyebrows in the centre of the forehead. Many Western students imagine it somewhere on the forehead. Actually, the activation centre corresponding to this chakra is in the brain between the eyebrows, but *behind* the frontal bone. If concentration on Sahasrara is correct, it is not difficult to perceive the beats in Ajna Chakra as well as in Sahasrara. It is best to turn the eyes up towards this imaginary point between the eyebrows. This position of the eyes must be maintained all throughout the Laya yoga or Kriya yoga exercises to be described later.

Some authors do not hesitate to identify this chakra with the pineal gland, long thought to be the seat of the soul. This minute gland, only eight millimetres long, is quite mysterious and even today its functions are not known. Some other authors do not hesitate to identify it with the famous 'third eye', but these considerations have an academic rather than a practical interest. What matters to us is that Ajna Chakra represents an essential meeting-place from a pranic viewpoint. Sushumna sends one of its terminal branches to it. Ida and Pingala have their origin in the nostrils but they go straight to Ajna Chakra. Therefore this crossing-point is one of the most important after Muladhara Chakra.

Ajna Chakra is sometimes called 'Siva Netra', meaning Siva's eye, or Jnana Netra, the eye of wisdom. The activation of Ajna Chakra is reputed to awaken intuition. We believe that concentration on this centre and its resulting activation can develop intuition because this is the centre of integration of the entire cerebral activity and not only of the cortex, the seat of the intellect.

Ajna Chakra also gives access to Sahasrara Chakra. They both function together and their activation rests on the same principle: to make us conscious of the pulsations of the blood in the various parts of the brain, which increases vascularisation (to keep within the realm of physiologicalexplanations) and benefits the exercise of related faculties.

Sahasrara Chakra

Sahasrara is usually described after Ajna Chakra. We mention it only as a reminder since we dealt with it earlier as the polar chakra of Muladhara Chakra.

41 | The Awakening of the Chakras

In our description of the chakras we limited ourselves to the essentials which should be perfectly understood by now. No time was wasted in giving details of the number of petals and their colours, the 'deities' of the chakras, and so on, as this has been done at length by Avalon and others. We did not go beyond the practical notions which are indispensable when applying the techniques for the awakening or the conscious activation of the chakras.

Preliminaries
In order toavoid those mishaps which we liken to pranic short-circuits each student must first practise the asanas, followed by the appropriate pranayama before starting to activate the chakras. The asanas make the dense body permeable to prana. Pranayama supplies the necessary energy and completes the action of the asanas. The exercises may then be performed without danger.

What does this practice consist of?
The student must sit in the lotus or siddhasana posture with the back of his hand resting on his knee in Jnana Mudra; he will gradually bring the energy of the 'species' pole back to the 'individual' pole, passing through all the energy centres on the way. In the techniques described below, concentration does not take place on the centre corresponding to Sushumna, but on the organs of resonance of these chakras. It is infinitely easier to be conscious of the resonance organs of the chakras than of the centres in the spine or in the Manomaya Kosha. The basic pranayama to activate the chakras as described in the present exercise has long been a well-kept secret: it is the pranayama square, which has the advantage of safeguarding the student against any excess of breath retention and of establishing the perfect balance between Prana and Apana so essential to these exercises. Consequently the practice of chakra activation can only be started after gaining complete mastery over the technique of the pranayama square (see p. 125). It is important to repeat the OM with the rhythm of the heartbeats during the whole exercise. The OM serves as a metronome while practising.

Awakening Muladhara Chakra

The student performs Mula Bandha and becomes aware of Apana energy; that is, he thinks of the excretory function of the organism situated in Muladhara. By continuing to concentrate on Muladhara and on Mula Bandha he also evokes the dynamic of the species which is expressed in the form of sexuality. He may evoke this power which for milillions of years has brought together innumerable couples who with- out interruption have transmitted life down to us. What matters is to be able to perceive this power as impersonal, as beyond the individual. For the individual it was important, of course, that his father should meet his mother. For the species this was a very minor detail. Thanks to sexual attraction the work of the species goes on and its continuation is ensured.

In Mula Bandha do not forget to contract the internal as well as the external sphincter. During the whole exercise the eyes are turned towards Ajna Chakra and breathing is regular. In the pranayama square the concentration is maintained for at least one minute.

The mere fact that we think of Muladhara Chakra already establishes a direct link between the centres of consciousness of Sahasrara Chakra, the brain and the root chakra. Mula Bandha and Asvini Mudra reinforce this link and intensify the current. Kriya yoga exercises reach this objective with great intensity. But thanks to yoga techniques, a very special process takes place in the student's organism. Apana Vayu is that particular form of prana which is manifested in the human body as excretory energy; Apana usually moves towards the outside in order to reject the impurities of the body, and almost always towards the lower part of the body – urination, defaecation, ejaculation, menstruation and childbirth, with the exception of perspiration and exhalation. Inhalation is performed by Prana Vayu; exhalation depends on Apana Vayu. By holding your breath you control both Prana Vayu and Apana Vayu provided that you practise Mula Bandha at the same time.

After practising this pranayama for a while (breath retention with Jalandhara and Mula Bandha combined), Apana Vayu is stimulated in Muladhara Chakra where it creates a strong pranic current, sometimes manifesting itself as a vibration clearly perceptible during rather prolonged breath retentions. The energising current which is created there tends automatically to rise along Sushumna in the direction of Sahasrara Chakra, meeting the various intermediary chakras on the way.

This process must be guided consciously by the yogi and the ascent

Plan of Chakra Activation

Activated Chakra	Bandha	Type of Pranayama	Organ of Resonance (mental concentration object)
Individual Pole Sahasrara Chakra		Pranayama Square	Perceive blood pulsations in the brain, at top of skull. Mentally draw all body forces there.
Ajna Chakra		Pranayama Square	Feel pulsations in the brain behind the frontal bone in the middle of the forehead.
Vishuddha Chakra		Pranayama Square	Concentrate on the throat (tongue, glottis, vocal cords). Imagine OM during the pranayama square.
Anahata Chakra	Jalandhara Bandha	Pranayama Square	Concentrate on the heart area. Perceive heartbeats. Think of blood circulation in the entire body.
Chandra Chakra	Jalandhara Bandha	Pranayama Square	Concentrate above and left of navel (spleen and pancreas area). Think of the energy of assimilation.
Surya Chakra	Jalandhara Bandha	Pranayama Square	Concentrate above and right of the navel (liver area). Think of the energy of assimilation.
Nabhi or Manipura Chakra	Jalandhara Bandha	Pranayama Square	Concentrate on the area of the navel. If possible, perceive blood pulsations there. Think of the energy of assimilation.
Svadisthana Chakra	Jalandhara Bandha + Asvini Mudra	Pranayama Square	During perineum contraction, concentrate on sensations perceived at the base of penis or clitoris. Think of sexual dynamism.
Muladhara Chakra Species Pole	Jalandhara Bandha + Mula Bandh	Pranayama Square	Concentrate on the zone activated by the contraction of the two anal sphincters and of perineum. Think of the species dynamism.

must be helped and accelerated by appropriate exercises. This prana ascent is called Pranuttana. Traditional treatises describe the resultant sensations as like a tingling or like hot steam spreading along the spine. This sensation is the most elementary and initial stage of the awakening chakras, manifested by the creation of centres of consciousness all along the spine, and particularly by the perception of light at certain levels.

Pranuttana continues with mental concentration on the successive chakras as described in the detailed plan p.221.

Activation is therefore performed in an upward direction, from the species pole in the sacrum towards the individual pole in the brain.

Concentration on these two basic chakras must not frighten those who have taken a vow of chastity. This exercise will allow them a more complete and easier sublimation of the energy of these centres by returning to the centre of the individual in Sahasrara Chakra.

Svadishana Chakra
There is no change at all in posture or breathing and the student remains in the pranayama square. He stops Mula Bandha and proceeds to Asvini Mudra with contraction of the perineum and of the base of the penis for men or of the clitoris for women. It is enough to remain perfectly conscious of these movements for about one minute before proceeding to the next chakra.

Nabhi (or Manipura Chakra)
Release the anal sphincter. During this whole phase concentrate on the navel and feel the blood pulsations (abdominal aorta) with possibly a contraction of the abdominal wall towards the end of the retention. Try to make mental perception penetrate that part of the abdomen around the navel and perceive the assimilatory energy which transforms food into the body's substance.

Surya and Chandra Chakras
The same technique and the same recommendations apply as above, but consciousness should move to the right of and above the navel towards the liver. Then repeat the process to the left towards the pancreas and the spleen.

Anahata Chakra
The pranayama square should be continued. What is essential here is to perceive the heartbeats. These pulsations must be slow and strong; if they become superficial and the heart races, this indicates that the retentions are too long or unsuitable for the student. Finally, while continuing to perceive the centre of the heartbeats, that is to say the heart area, the pulsations must be felt to shake the whole body.

Vishuddha Chakra
Pranayama square without bandhas; be conscious of the entire throat area. Imagine the silent OM, but feel the vocal chords almost in motion as though actually chanting OM. Breathe slowly and consciously while concentrating on the throat, especially on the glottis. Be conscious of the tongue and especially of its root.

Ajna Chakra
Pranayama square without bandhas. Throughout the exercise the eyes are turned towards Ajna, but perception of this particular point was a little confused during concentration on the lower centres. Now we must be aware of the beats and pulsations behind the frontal bone, in the middle of the forehead. Concentrate on this as long as possible. Be well aware of the air passing through the nostrils and imagine that through them (Ida and Pingala) energy is being taken in; direct it towards the centre of the beats, the point in Ajna Chakra.

Sahasrara Chakra
We have now reached the individual pole. The technique is the same as for Ajna Chakra, but it is necessary to feel all the forces in the body reaching that spot in the middle of the head where the pulsations of the blood are perceived and from there you must feel them radiating throughout the body. Imagine that the head is filled with light and warmth.

Imagine also the OM, OM, OM to the rhythm of the blood's pulsations. Be aware of the unity of consciousness and the entire body; such perception should give joy. The exercise may then be repeated, beginning at Muladhara Chakra, or it may be interrupted.

Additional instructions
The essential condition of this exercise is awareness of the various parts of the body, the inner concentration on the organs which serve

as projections of the chakras involved. The centre, or the real chakra, is automatically activated in Sushumna in association with Sahasrara. Perceptions become more and more precise with practice. Reaction on the spiritual centre may create colours, but these are not indispensable The sable for the success of the exercise; in order to avoid any possibility of suggestion, no mention is made here of what colour or colours may be perceived, and in themselves they are unimportant anyway.

This exercise gives control over Manomaya Kosha and Vijnamaya Kosha as well as over pranamaya Kosha. This is the point of fusion of the so-called 'physical' yoga and the so-called 'mental' yoga or Raja yoga, the two being inseparable. Four levels of existence can be integrated, thanks to pranayama. As the student improves, this exercise of meditation on the chakras and their awakening (or consciousness) will fill him with joy. Thus Anandamaya Kosha gradually penetrates all the other koshas. This joy is both a reward and the proof of correct and beneficial practice. It will give the student dynamic health and serenity, sheltering him from the turbulence and the inevitable tribulations of life.

Length of the exercise
An average pranayama square lasts at least half a minute, so nine chakras will occupy about five minutes. A minute of three complete cycles is necessary and this represents at least a quarter of an hour of practice. Actually, a serious-minded Western student should double that time, and in India the exercise may continue for two hours. For less than half an hour it may be performed without reservations, but a whole hour's exercise may have special physical or psychic effects for each individual and that is why the presence of a qualified guide is indispensable. However, with self-observation a student should be able to feel how far he may go, provided he practises regularly every day.

42 | Pranuttana, the Ascent of Prana

There is a great variety of tantric and other exercises for the activation of the chakras. They are often very complicated, requiring much time and also the supervision of a qualified guide who can adapt them to each individual.

The following technique has several advantages: (1) it is free from any Hindu or other ideology; (2) it can be safely practiced by a Westerner; (3) it does not require too much time. It is, however, authentic and classic. As with the postures, it is not necessarily the most acrobatic position that is the most effective. It is possible to design a well balanced yoga session, well adapted to Western needs, by using only simple asanas. It is useless to start practising kriyas if one does not regularly practice the pranayama exercises described above, particularly those designed to purify the nadis (alternate and rhythmic breathing). It is essential to practise Pranuttana in the lotus position or in siddhasana; no other position is suitable.

Preparation and interiorisation
Breathe calmly through both nostrils. Concentrate on the passage of the air through the nose and imagine that a warm vapour comes out of the nose during the prolonged exhalation. During inhalation imagine that luminous air is entering the nose and that this light is prana. This is not far from the scientific truth, as light is one of the forms of energy in the atmosphere.

Pranuttana
The ascent of prana occurs mainly during exhalation. Carry out Mula Bandha while concentrating on Muladhara Chakra and imagine warmth at the sacrum. During exhalation imagine the energy rising up the spine like warm sap in a tree and guide this energy to Sahasrara. During the whole exhalation imagine OM (one single, long OM). The mind has to be completely absorbed in this pranayama. During inhalation concentrate again on the OM. Let the inhaled air penetrate you and guide the prana first to Sahasrara and then towards Muladhara. The breath should not be held. Exhalation should either be as long as

inhalation or, preferably, twice as long, if that does not cause fatigue. Mula Bandha may be relaxed during inhalation if it should prove too tiring to hold during the entire exercise. Continue for at least five minutes, so that the mind can become completely absorbed in the act of breathing and you will really feel warmth all along the spine.

The mental image aids in the creation of this warmth. The yogis imagine a brazier of glowing coals in the triangle at the bottom of the spine. During inhalation this fire is fanned by imaginary bellows. Thus the yogi sends prana along Sushumna and makes it pass through all the chakras. Long and persistent practice is needed to achieve these results. The final aim is the complete mastery of prana in the body and, via the chakras, the mastery of Manomaya Kosha, the activity of the mind.

Thus we begin to see the aim of pranayama, which is one of the necessary steps leading the student towards the most subtle regions of his innermost being. Pranayama builds the solid basis for a total integration of all the koshas and their activity. In any case, even when it does not awaken the chakras, this exercise gives the student increased vitality and an intensified psycho-physical dynamism which he can use at will. It calms the nerves, gives him a new serenity and also helps him to develop his powers of concentration.

We now have ample techniques at our fingertips, all the details that can be given in writing without danger to anyone. How should we use these techniques in a progressive and co-ordinated manner? There will be no problems if the following rules are remembered:

1 Respect the ethical and dietetic rules for a healthy life.
2 Practise the other techniques of Hatha yoga regularly, particularly a daily session of asanas, not forgetting the sun worship. These are the best preparation for pranayama and the best defence against any possible risk in its practice. The asanas make the body receptive to the pranic forces and favour the absorption and correct distribution of prana in the body. They enable the student to remain motionless for a long time and effortless in an asana which is suitable for a pranayama session.
3 Use the conscious control of prana during the practice of the asanas. While breathing, always concentrate on the breath and on those parts of the body affected by the particular asana. Balance prana and apana during the whole session, making sure that inhalation and exhalation are of exactly the same length. Practise Ujjayi (the partial blockage of the glottis) during the whole asana session.
4 When you feel the marvellous effect of pranayama on your body and your psyche, you might be tempted to consider the asanas as secondary and to practise them only 'to maintain the suppleness of the body', or even to neglect them completely. This would be a grave error and the sign of a total lack of understanding of pranayama and its applications to all phases, both physical and mental, of yoga. In India, the masters do not allow their pupils to reduce the practice of the asanas when they pass to pranayama, but rather make them intensify it.
5 Advance slowly in the practice of the techniques of pranayama, especially in those exercises which require breath retention. At the beginning be wise: obey all instructions carefully, particularly the gradual increase in the length of retention.
6 The essential element in pranayama is the concentration of the mind on the exercises. There is no pranayama without concentration. Pranayama is part of Hatha yoga, but it also belongs to Raja

yoga, the yoga of control of the mind.

7 The passing to a higher stage may occur when the lungs and the body are perfectly at ease during the preceding exercises and when the mind is ready to concentrate on the breath with a minimum of distraction.

8 You must, however, accept distractions as inevitable. When they occur, immediately lead the mind back to the exercise. Only long practice enables you to absorb your mind completely in pranayama or the asanas.

9 Establish your programme of progressive practice (see below for suggestions) but do not fix a time limit for passing from one stage to the next.

10 In pranayama, more than in anything else, regular daily practice leads to success and is the best protection against possible dangers. If one day you are really unable to practise, do not let the day go by without carrying out some complete yogic respirations and concentrate on your breathing from time to time.

Suggested programmes

The following programmes are suitable for the majority of Westerners. Before each session these conditions must be fulfilled:

1 Empty the bladder and, if possible, the bowels.
2 Clean the nose by practising neti, drying the nostrils carefully.
3 If one nostril remains blocked in spite of neti, use one of the clearing processes described in this book (see p 67).
4 Practise in the open air if possible, or at least in a well ventilated room, heated in the winter.
5 Except when instructions are given to the contrary (as in Sitali and Sitkari, for instance), always breathe through the nose. This applies to inhalation as well as to exhalation.
6 Immobilise the tongue at the top of the gums of the upper front teeth or bend it back against the soft palate. Swallow your saliva, if necessary.
7 Practise with your eyes shut or almost shut if you are looking at the tip of your nose (tratak).
8 Take up your posture with care: see that the spine is in the correct position. Relax the face, the shoulders, the arms, the forearms and the hands as much as possible during exercises.

9   The nose is not a suction pump. The only noise which may be audible is that produced by the braking of the air in the glottis and not the friction of air in the nose. The nostrils must be in a position to allow correct inhalation.

These preliminary conditions apply to all stages of pranayama.

First stage
1   Before beginning pranayama it is essential to concentrate on the respiration and to shorten and slow the breath (see p. 56). Practice this concentration for two to five minutes according to the time available. Do not make the sessions too long at the beginning.
2   After concentration comes the necessary purification of the nadis through the practice of Nadi Sodhana (see p. 56)), alternate respiration without breath retention. Devote the same amount of time to Nadi Sodhana as you did to concentration. Always practise with the abdomen controlled (see p. 66).
3   Right from the start, if you have enough time you may practise Prana Mudra (see p. 97).
4   Also right from the beginning, you may practise pranic recharging (see p. 124), either when you have a moment to spare or even in bed, if you have no other free time.

At the end of each pranayama session relax for one to three minutes (or longer, if possible) according to the time available.

Second stage
As soon as the preliminary conditions are fulfilled, start your session with concentration (1 above) and Nadi Sodhana (2 above) for two to five minutes altogether. When you feel that you are concentrating well, change Nadi Sodhana into Anuloma Viloma, that is to say, add a breath retention. It is not necessary to measure its length. Devote at least five minutes to Anuloma Viloma. During these retentions you must strictly respect the rules for Kumbhaka (see p. 82). If the retention lasts more than ten seconds Jalandhara Bandha becomes obligatory (see p. 133)). Jalandhara Bandha and Anuloma Viloma will allow you to train your lungs progressively in breath retention with complete safety

Without changing your session you can progressively introduce rhythm into your practice, say after two or three more weeks (see p. 88). You can also add the pranayama square to your practice. Practise pranic recharging, possibly at times other than your session, as well as Prana Mudra. This programme may be divided into two daily sessions of from ten to fifteen minutes each.

Third stage
At this level you need two sessions of pranayama daily. One session in the morning, or, if not possible, before lunch and a second one before the evening meal. Now the sessions can start directly with Anuloma Viloma.

The pranayama square follows and should last about five minutes. Now add Kapalabhati (without alternate breathing) to your practice. Read attentively all the information given in the relevant section (see pp. 149–156) and practise slowly at first. Let speed develop with practice. Once you get up speed, do not go beyond 120 expulsions per minute. Practise for five minutes, rest period included. Kapalabhati quickly tires the abdominal muscles and this is a safeguard against the enthusiasm of the beginner.

After reasonable practice of Kapalabhati I (two or three weeks) you may move on to Kapalabhati 11 (see p. 154) with alternate breathing. Prana Mudra will close the session.

Fourth stage
Two sessions per day. They may be of the same pattern as those of the previous stage. Kapalabhati should be practised for about two minutes, with both nostrils open. After a rest period - in the posture - during which complete yogic breathing with abdominal control should be practised, Kapalabhati with alternate breathing may be started. After another rest you may practise Bhastrika. Otherwise keep to the exercises of the third stage.

Fifth stage
Three sessions per day. Kapalabhati for two minutes (with alternate breathing). Bhastrika for three minutes. Then Surya Bedha Kumbhaka. Anuloma Viloma with prolonged retentions. Practise Asvini Mudra at odd moments. Mula Bandha and Ujjayi.

Sixth stage
Three sessions per day. For the first two sessions: programme as above. Then add the bandhas to the practice of pranayama and of the as-

anas. During the third session devote a third of the available time to the exercises as above. The remaining two-thirds should be used for activation of the chakras, which crowns the practice of pranayarna (see pp. 219–224).

With the sixth stage we reach the limit of practice permissible in the West (or indeed anywhere else) without a qualified guide.

These programmes are, however, only suggestions and not a rigid framework. The length of each session and the moving on from one stage to the next are left to the discretion of the student. The reactions of his body and his mind will guide him. With the help of his trusted guru, common sense and good measure, the student will be successful.

Errors to be avoided

1 Never practise during the initial phase of digestion. While the moderate pranayama exercises may be done when the digestion is reasonably advanced (one or two hours after food), exercises with prolonged retention may only be done three hours after a meal at the earliest.
2 Always begin by cleansing the nostrils (neti and Kapalabhati will see to this).
3 Never practise with a sagging spine. It must be straight and upright.
4 Do not talk to anybody about your practice.
5 Do not change your programme constantly. Establish a routine and let your body and your lungs get used to it.
6 Do not skip the different stages. Haste does not pay in yoga.
7 Do not practise haphazardly according to your daily whim; keep to your programme.
8 Do not be timid. If you stick to the rules, the exercises described in this book are not dangerous.
9 If, in spite of everything, there has been an interruption in your practice, do not take up your training where you left off but follow again - more quickly this time - all the previous stages.
10 Never practise so much that you get tired. As soon as you begin to feel tired, interrupt the exercise and take up Shavasana.

ALSO AVAILABLE AT HARMONY PUBLISHING:

YOGA: *The Art of Adjusting* – Brian Cooper

This teaching manual is aimed at teachers and students of Hatha Yoga who wish to incorporate adjusting into their teaching practice. The Asanas of the primary series of the Astanga system are the basis for this manual. The principles of adjusting are explained to ensure adjustments are carried out safely and effectively. Each Asana is shown along with its detailed alignment, followed by clearly illustrated and beautifully photographed adjustments. Different styles of adjusting are shown including partner yoga and Thai Massage.

HATHA YOGA: *the report of a personnal experience* – Theos Bernards

About Theos Bernard:

His begins in the 1930s, when he was suffering from a severe attack of inflammatory rheumatism while studying at law school. In hospital he overheard the doctors say that he would not live. After weeks of suffering, his mother removed him, against the wishes of the doctors, and took on the task of nursing him back to health. Bernard was put on a strict vegetarian diet and spent time in the mountains of Arizona. Slowly he recovered, and during this time, from reading in his mother's large library of books on Eastern philosophy, he first saw the possibility that yoga would be his way to gaining both inner and outer strength. Through family connections he had a visit from his first Indian guru who explained to him that the Tantras had been revealed for the liberation of man in this dark age of the Kali Yuga. The guru left him with two sets of exercises, one for physical and one for mental health. And so began Bernard's daily practice of yoga.

Excerpt from the preface:

"In 1935, after the grand tour I submitted to a course of traditional training in Hatha Yoga, taking notes and making critical observations in order to appraise the results in the light of experience rather than of theory. I was, in fact, induced to make this practical trial of Yoga because of the disappointments I experienced in. connection with Yoga theory. The theories, about which there is an abundant literature, were confusing rather than informative regarding the practical content and discipline of Hatha Yoga. To this end I became the sincere disciple of a highly esteemed teacher and settled down at his retreat in the hills near Ranchi. Under his supervision and guidance I adhered to the rigid discipline imposed upon one who wishes to practice Hatha Yoga."